Moonbox

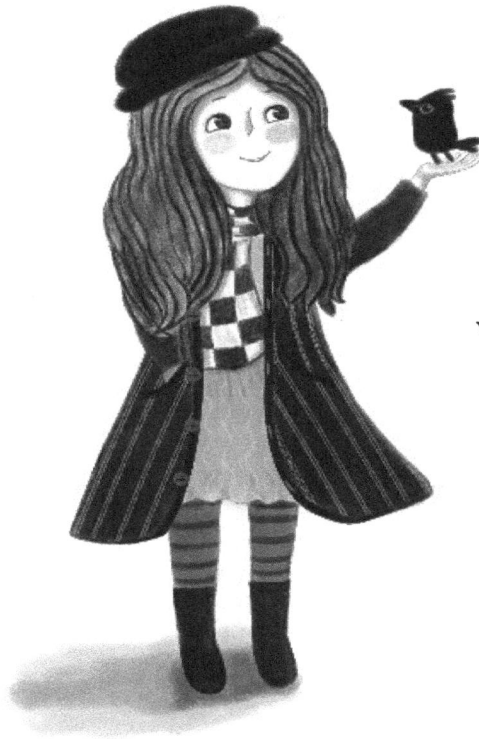

Written by
Liz Carruth

Illustrated by
Vrushali Sarwate

To contact the author: lizcarruth@gmail.com

Edited by: Elisabeth Carruth & Rebecca Clawson

Cover art, Layout, Illustrated by: Vrushali Sarwate

ISBN: 979-8-9857920-0-3

First printing, 2022

Diisclaimer: The information in this book is of the author's own research and made in good faith.
The author has tried to present all information as accurately and faithfully as possible. The information
therefore is not intended to diagnose, treat, or replace medical authority of doctors.

For my mother, my best friend.

Thank you for always believing in me.

Mama told me about the moon and her phases when I was young. When I couldn't let her go anywhere without me. I use to think it was this special bond we shared; a secret that only we knew.

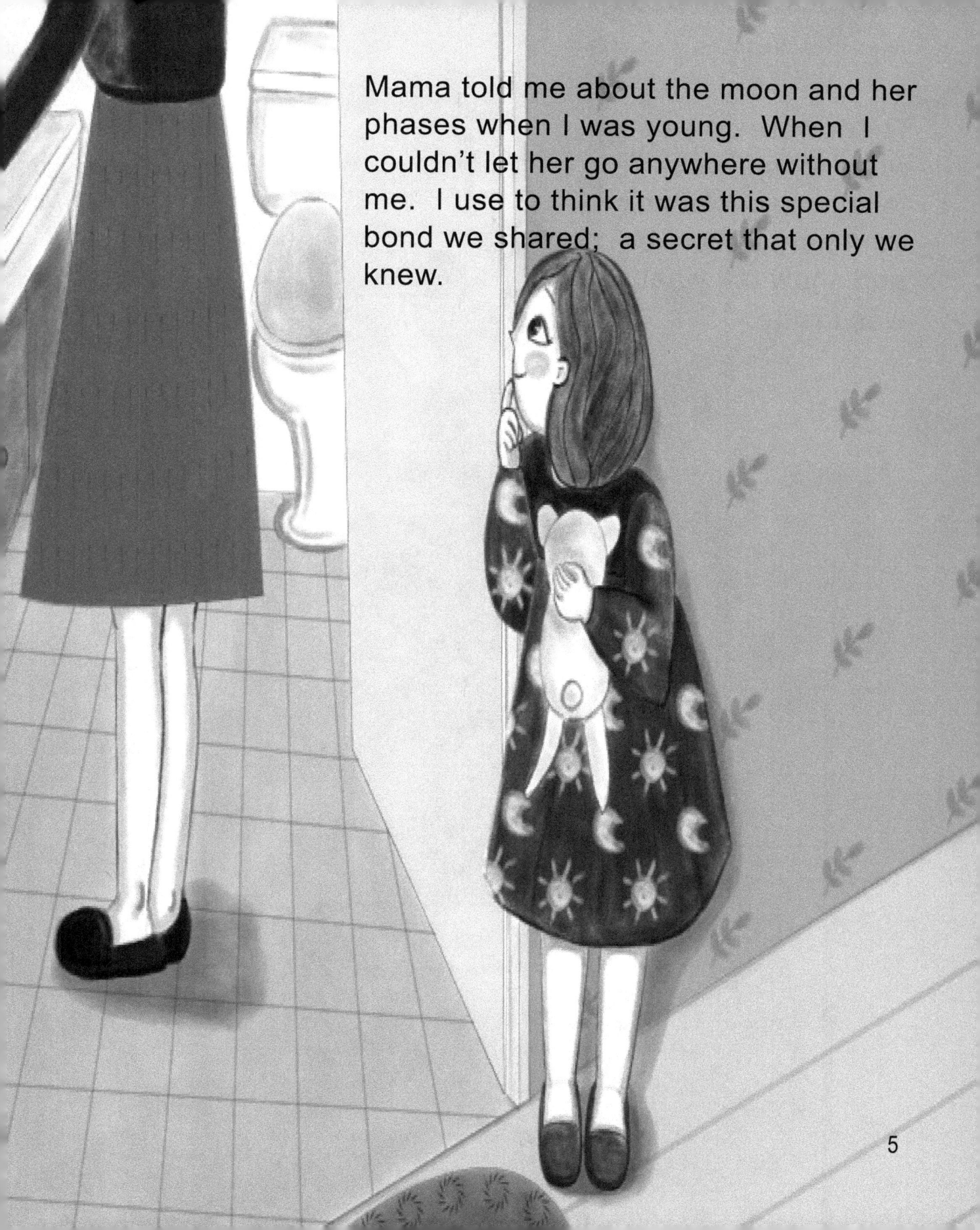

There were times
when Mama would
take her *special box*
from her top drawer
and show me what
was inside.

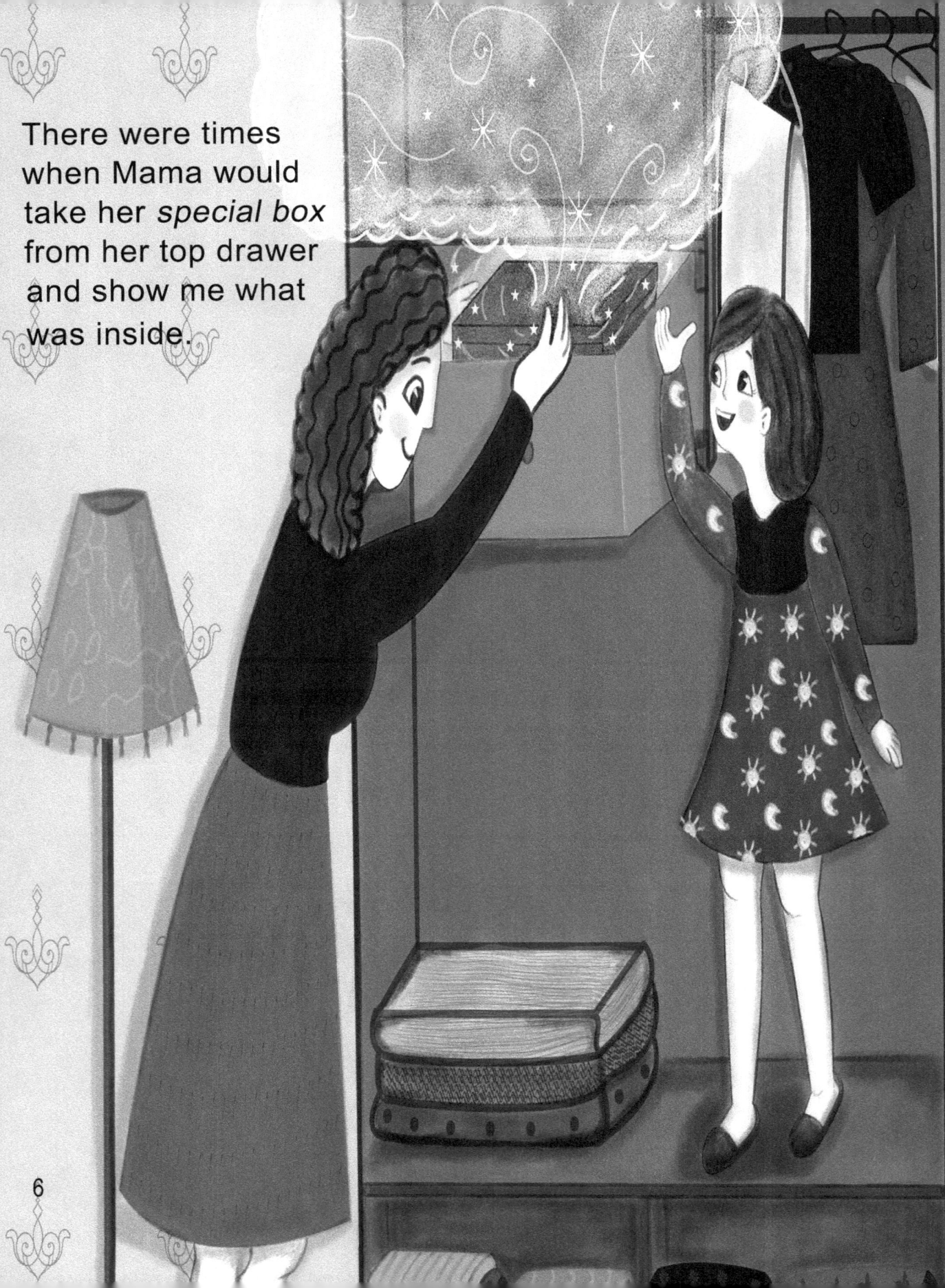

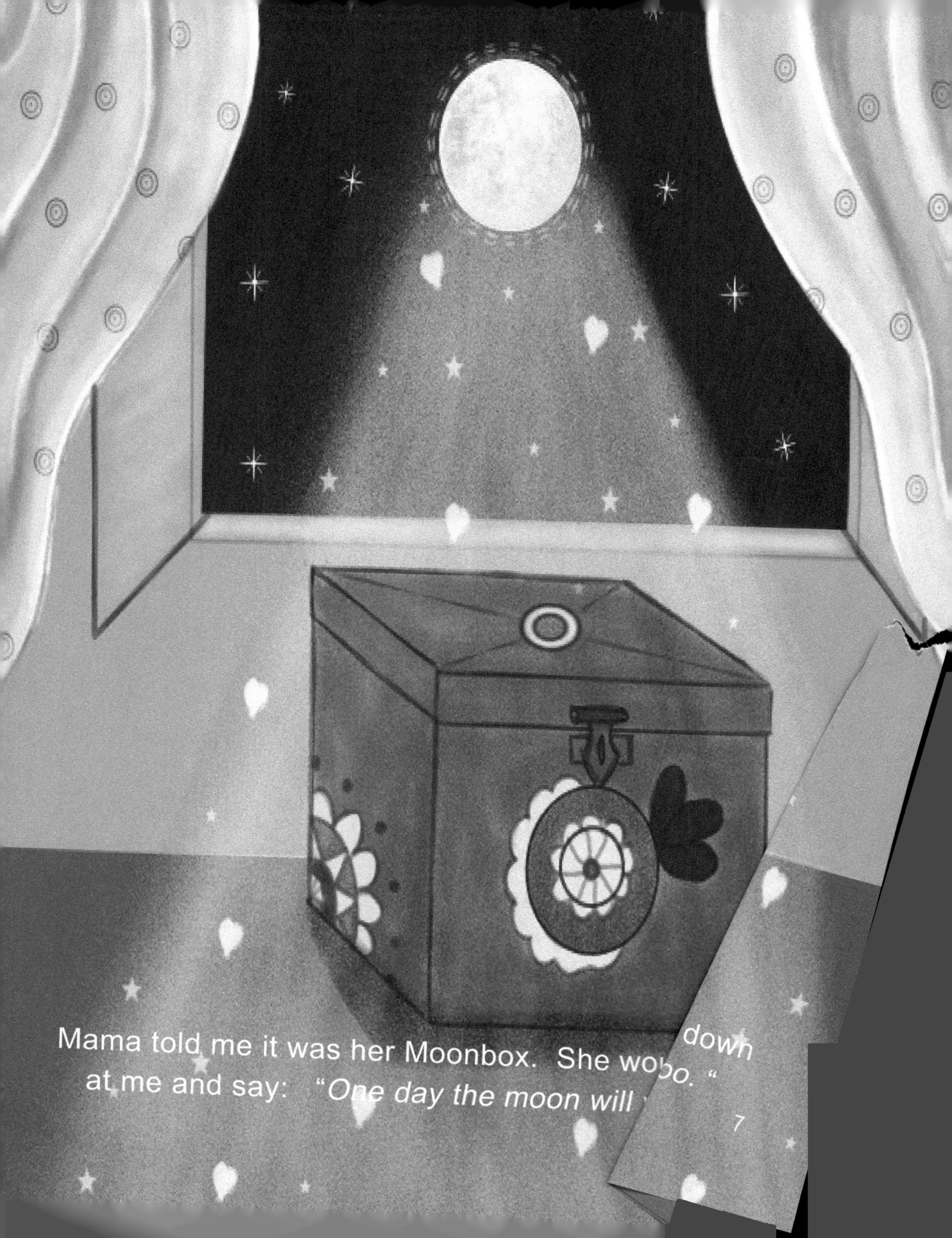

Mama told me it was her Moonbox. She wobo. " down
at me and say: "One day the moon will

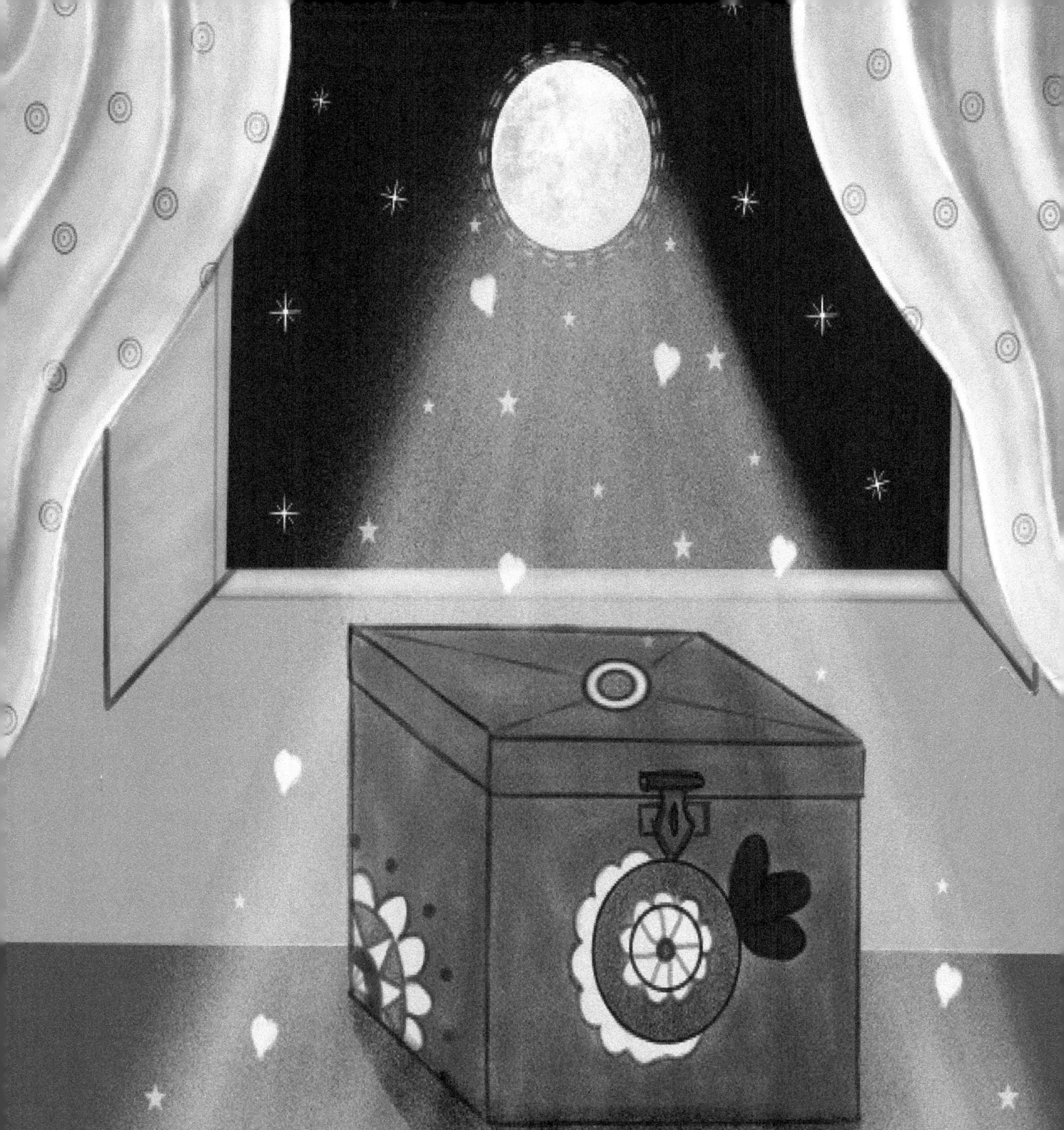

Mama told me it was her Moonbox. She would smile down
at me and say: "*One day the moon will visit you too.*"

7

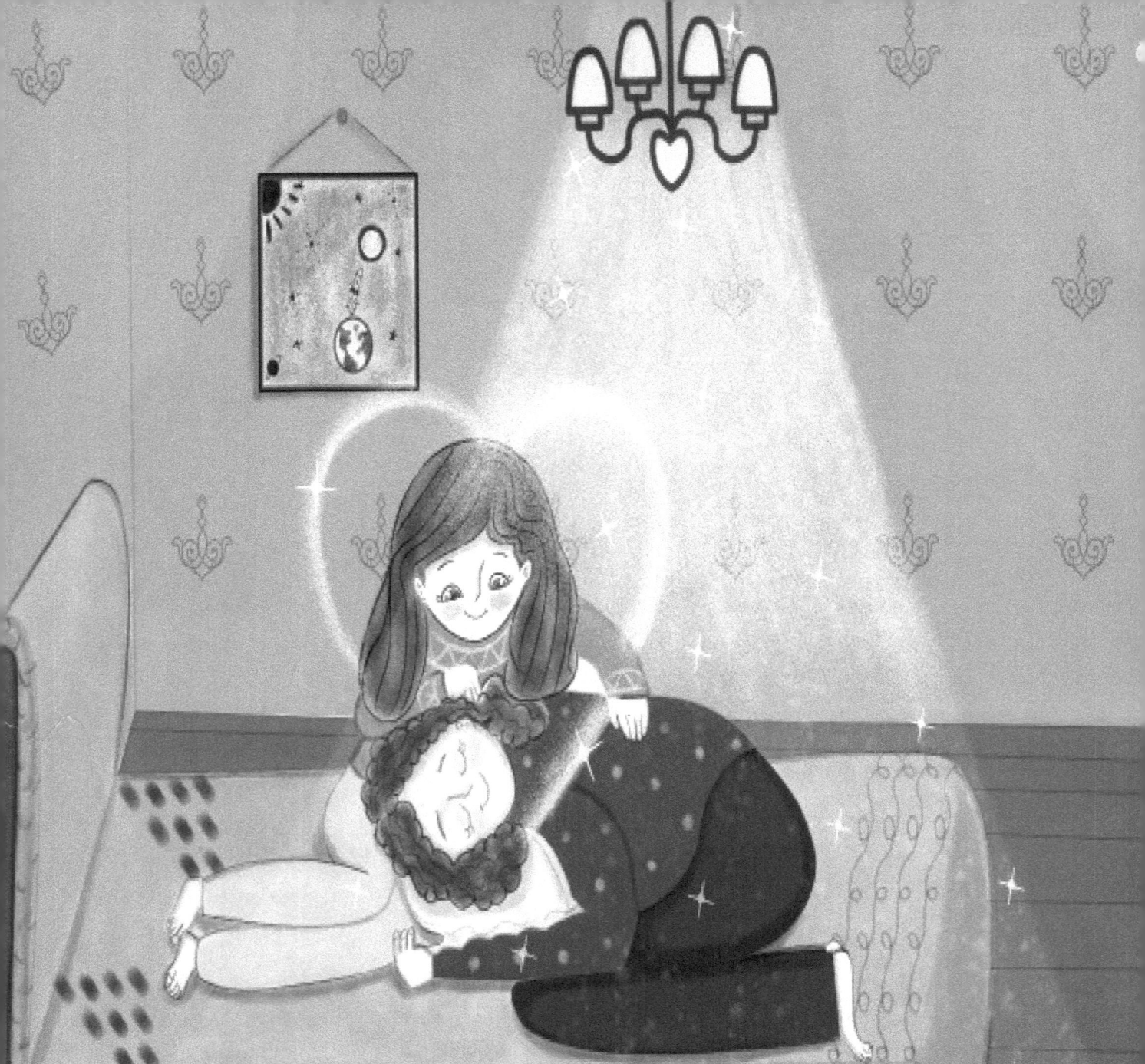

I didn't know what was happening or why but I knew something special had happened to Mama. It didn't happen very often but there were times when Mama was cranky or wanted to cuddle.

Sometimes I'd find Mama sneaking a snack or napping on the couch. Sometimes Mama would cry over everything. But most of the time Mama was happy.

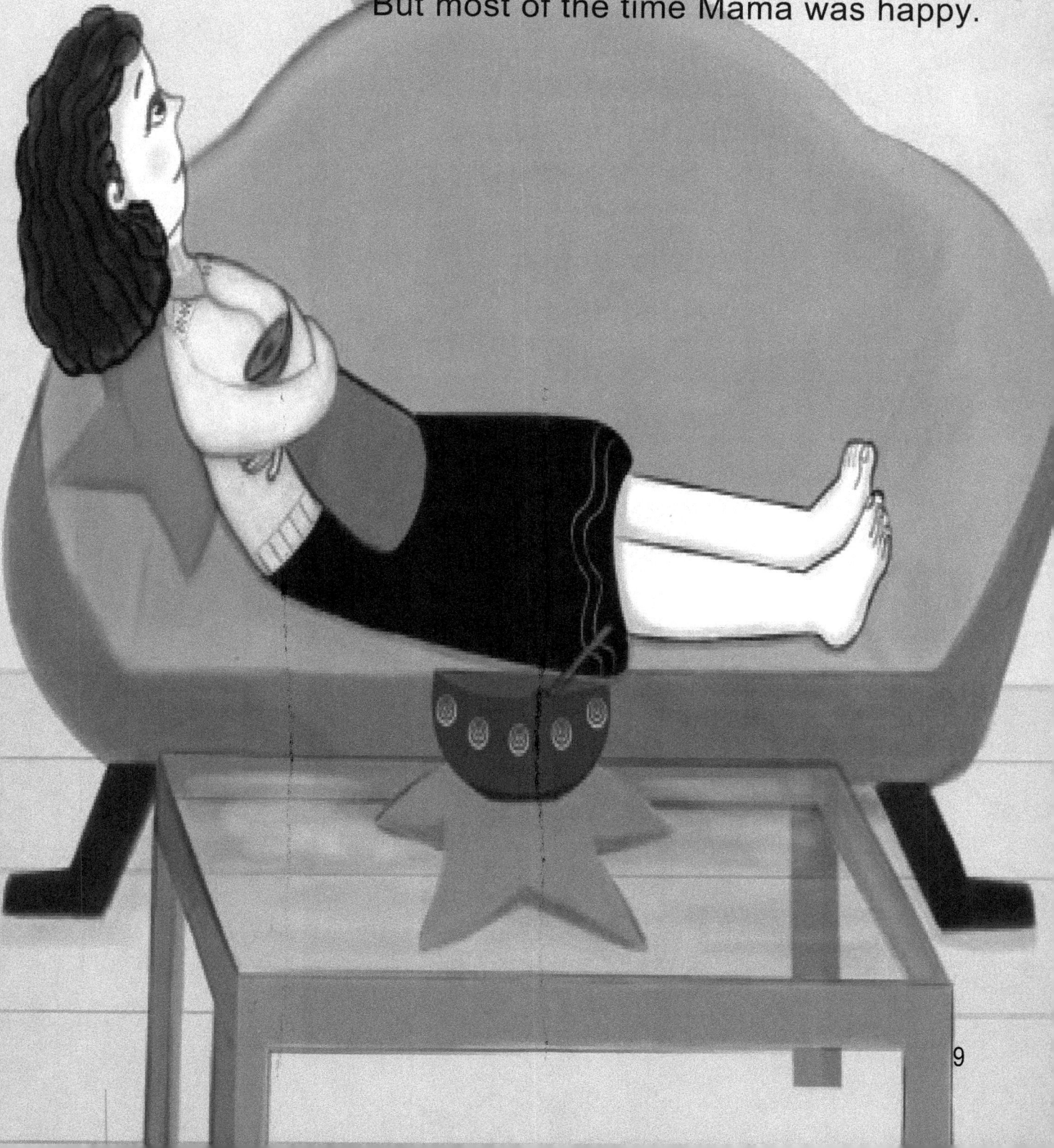

I used to love sorting Mama's Moonbox. Sometimes by size and color. Sometimes by what Mama liked most. Mama would smile down at me and say:

"*One day the moon will visit you too.*"
Mama never said when but I was glad someday I would have my own Moonbox to sort.

One day, as I was sorting Mama's Moonbox,
I asked: "Do all girls have a Moonbox?"
Mama paused, then said: "Yes!"

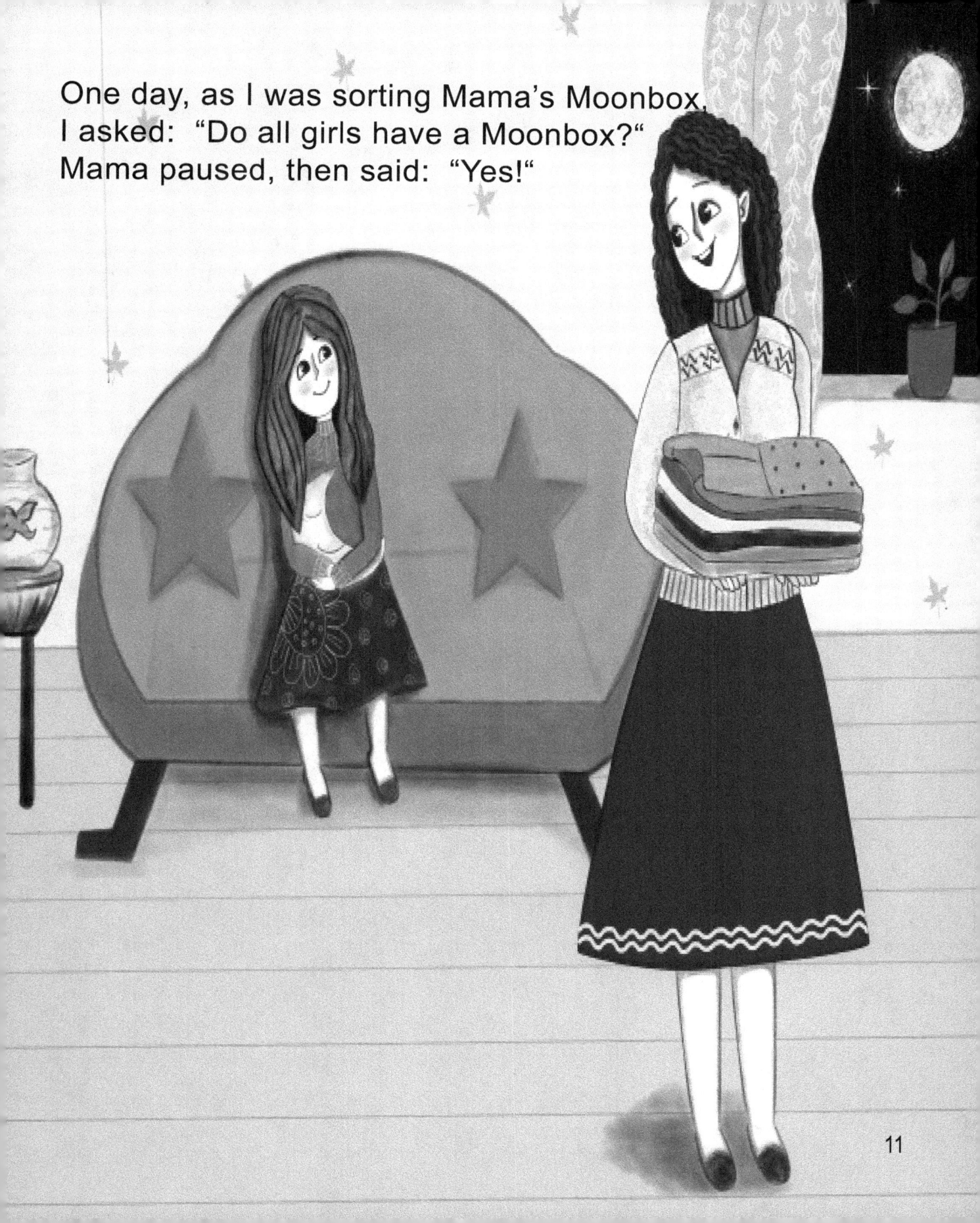

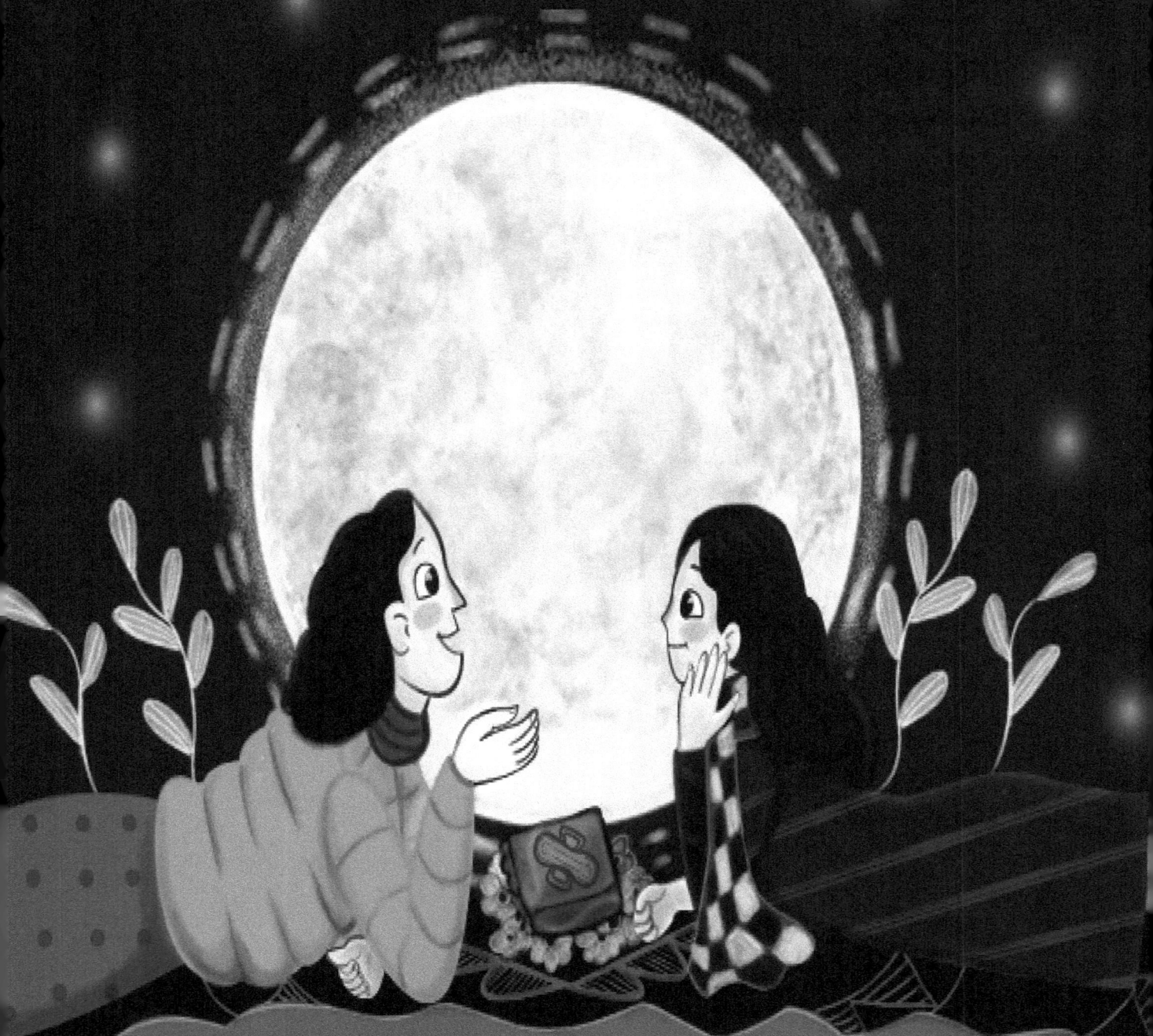

"Sometimes they are made with fabric and cloth like mine."
Mama held up a very colorful pad that had signs of much use.
Fabric "rags" are what girls have been using for a long time.
I like using cloth because it's natural and better for the earth.
We can dispose of the cloth when it's no longer usable. "

"Some girls have just a simple *cup* made from soft silicone.

Sometimes a Moonbox has rows of *cotton tampons* or natural *sea sponges*.

Sometimes a Moonbox is made with *disposable materials* like grocery store pads."

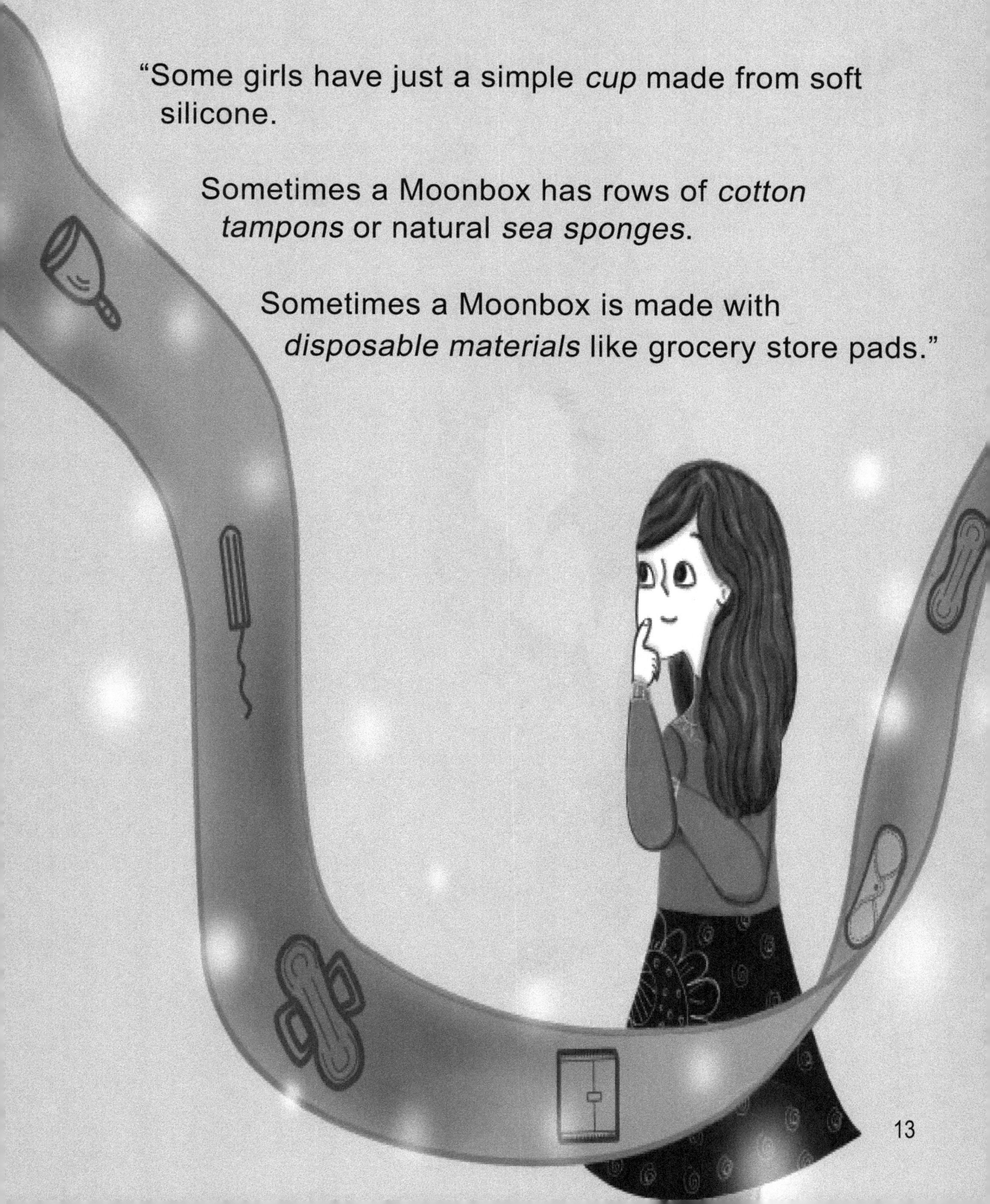

With much excitement Mama drew me to my feet
"So, yes! Every girl the moon has visited will have a
Moonbox." Mama hugged me. "It's a very special time in
a girl's life. It means you're a woman."

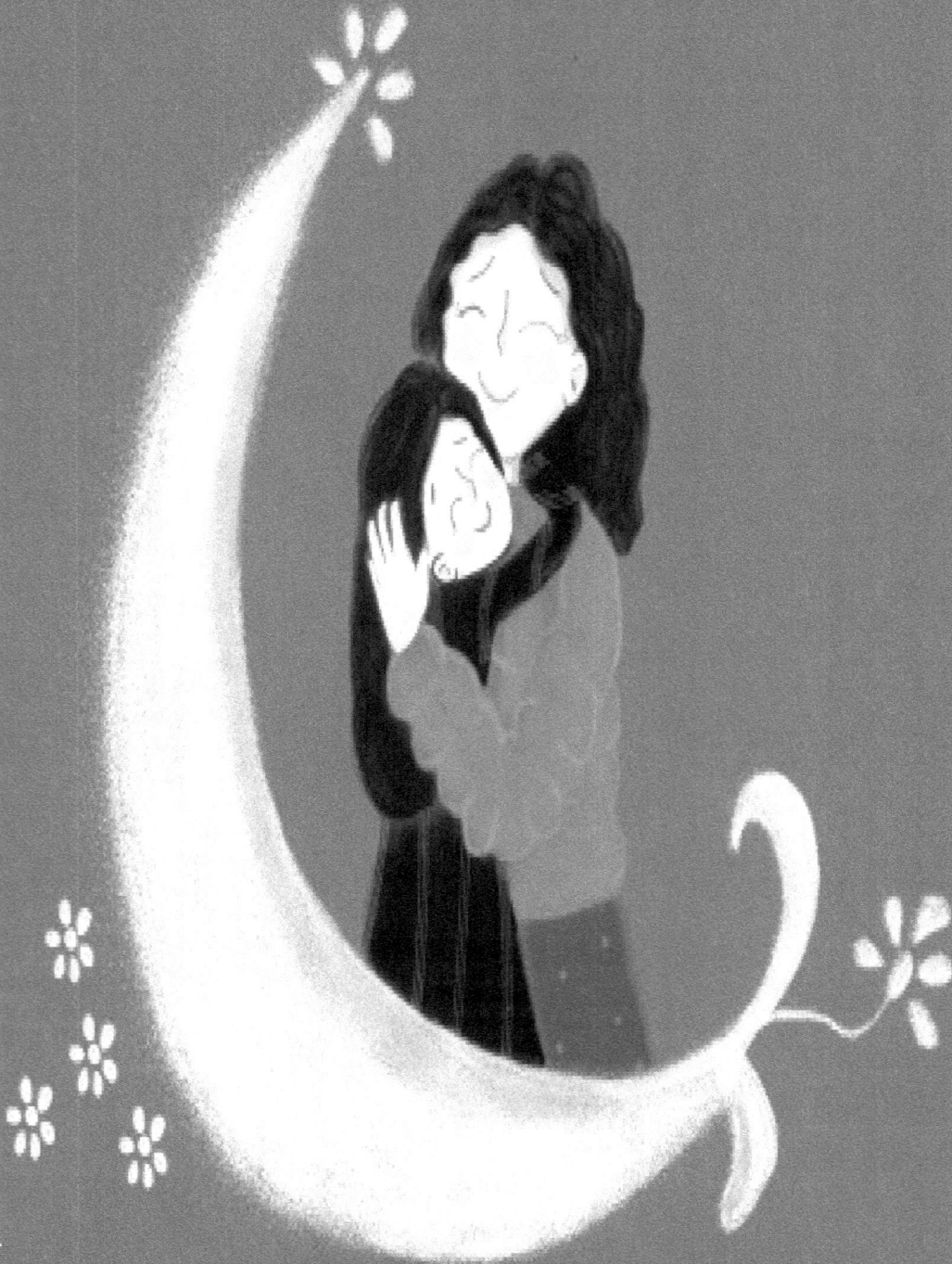

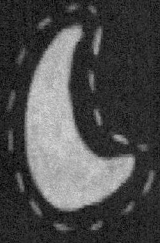

Mama and I looked to the sky and stared at the moon.
"Women are capable of doing anything!
Becoming anything!
A Moonbox is like everything else in life,
it's up to *you* what to put into it."

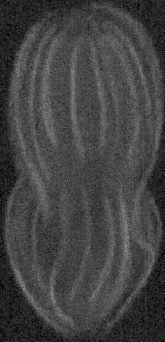

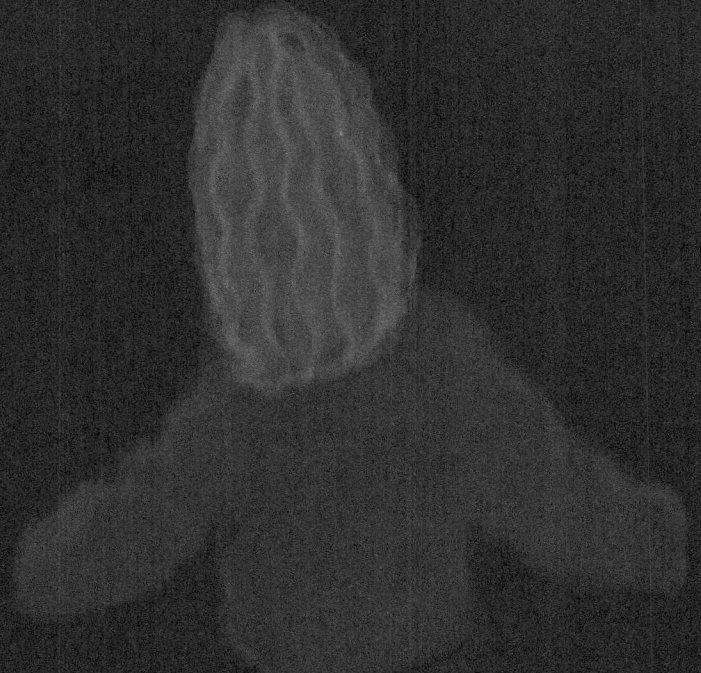

Sometimes I'd sit at my window and wonder when it will be time to open my own Moonbox.

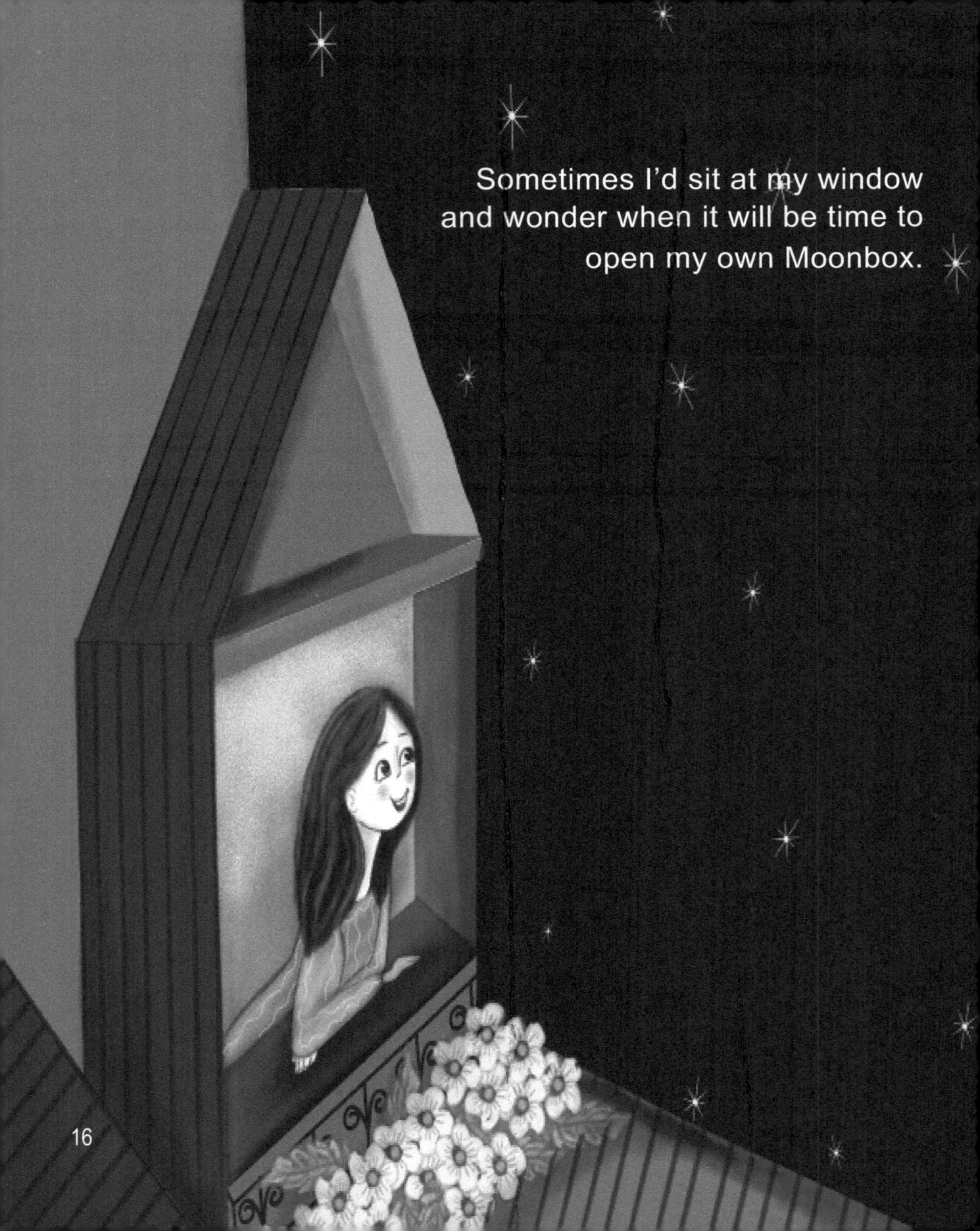

I remember asking Mama: "When will the moon visit me too?"

Mama smiled and knew just what to say.

Reaching for the bookcase Mama said:

"As you grow your body is doing amazing things."

Mama brought out a book on the body and she showed me what we look like on the inside.

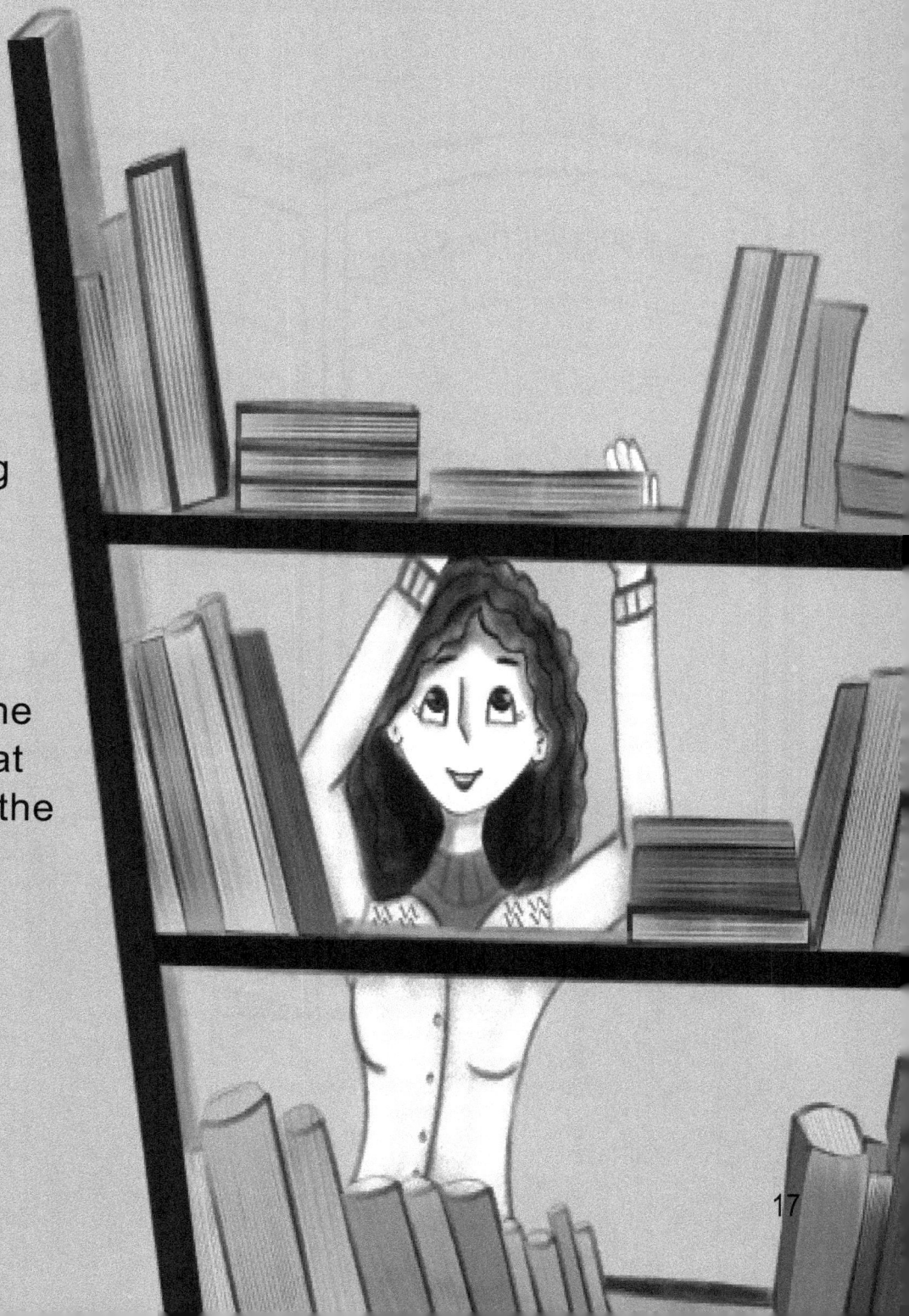

17

Pointing to the small bean shape on the page Mama said: "Inside these little ovaries live thousands of eggs and hormones. The eggs are only half of the materials needed to create life!"

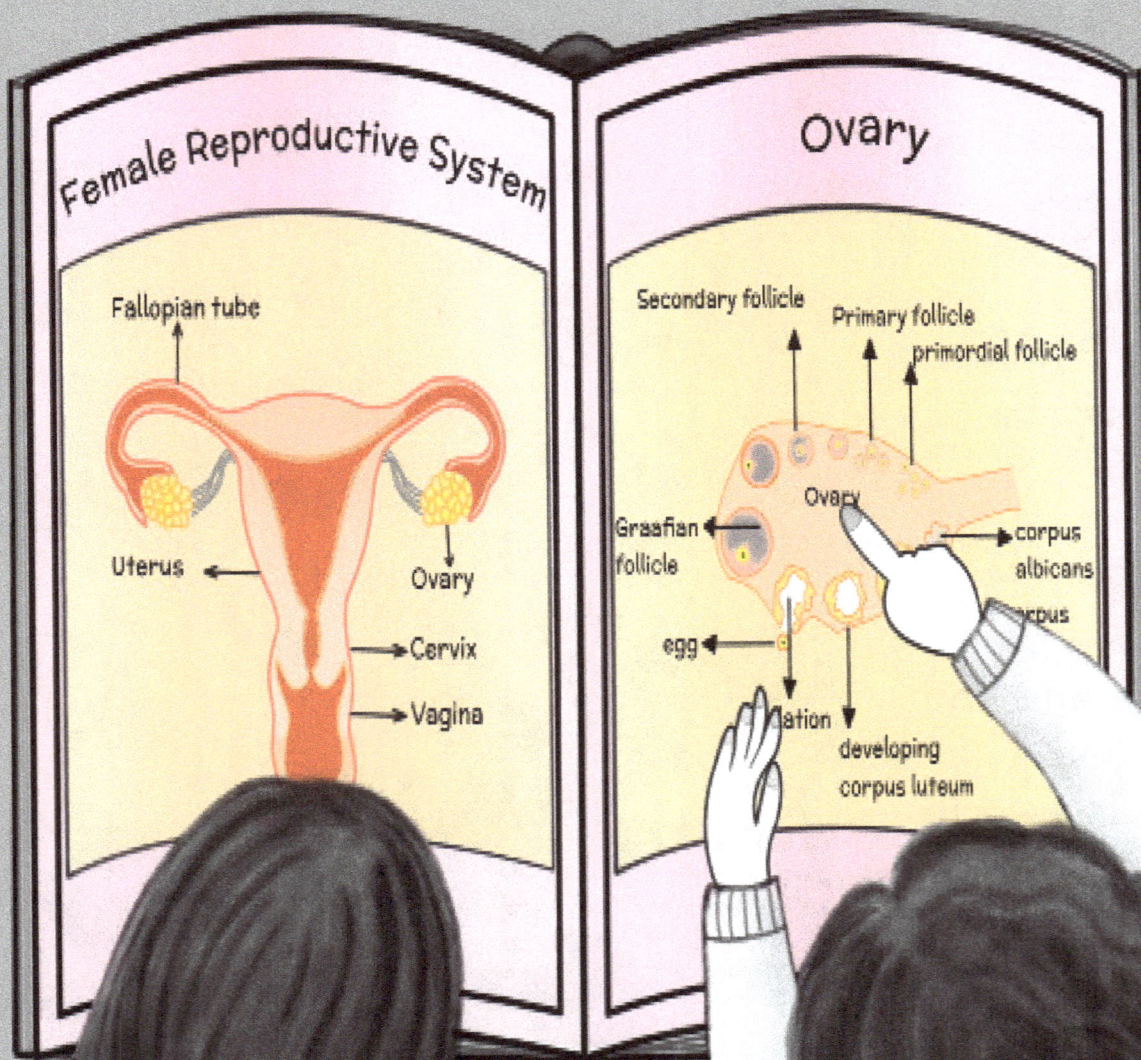

Female Reproductive System

Fallopian tube

Uterus

Ovary

Cervix

Vagina

Ovary

Secondary follicle

Primary follicle

primordial follicle

Graafian follicle

Ovary

corpus albicans

egg

developing corpus luteum

"Just as the moon waxes until it reaches its full phase, so do your body's hormones. These hormones tell the ovaries to release an egg. That egg only has a few days to become a baby."

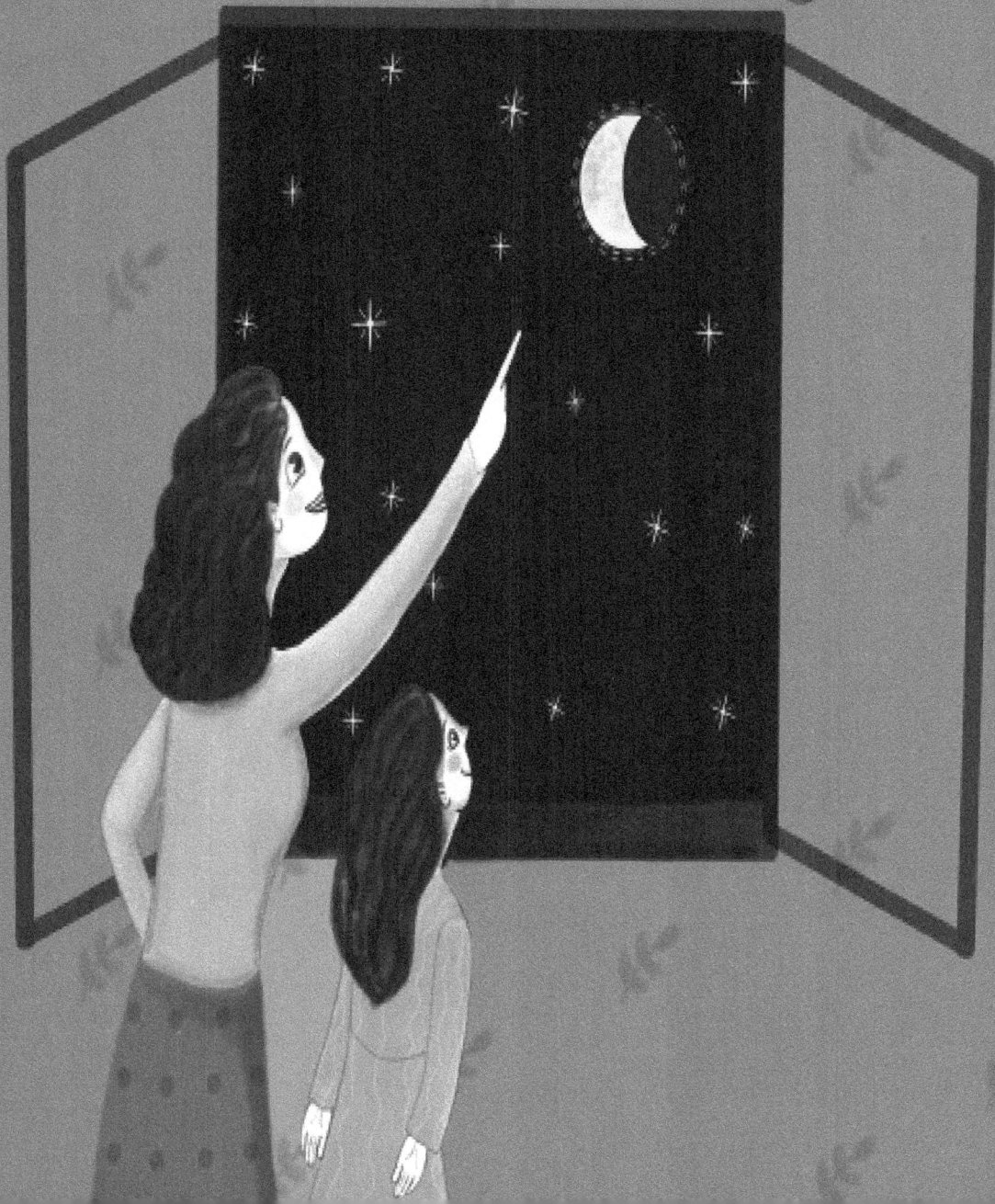

"The egg slowly travels down the fallopian tube to the uterus where the lining has been thickening to become a nourishing environment for if the egg were to become a baby."

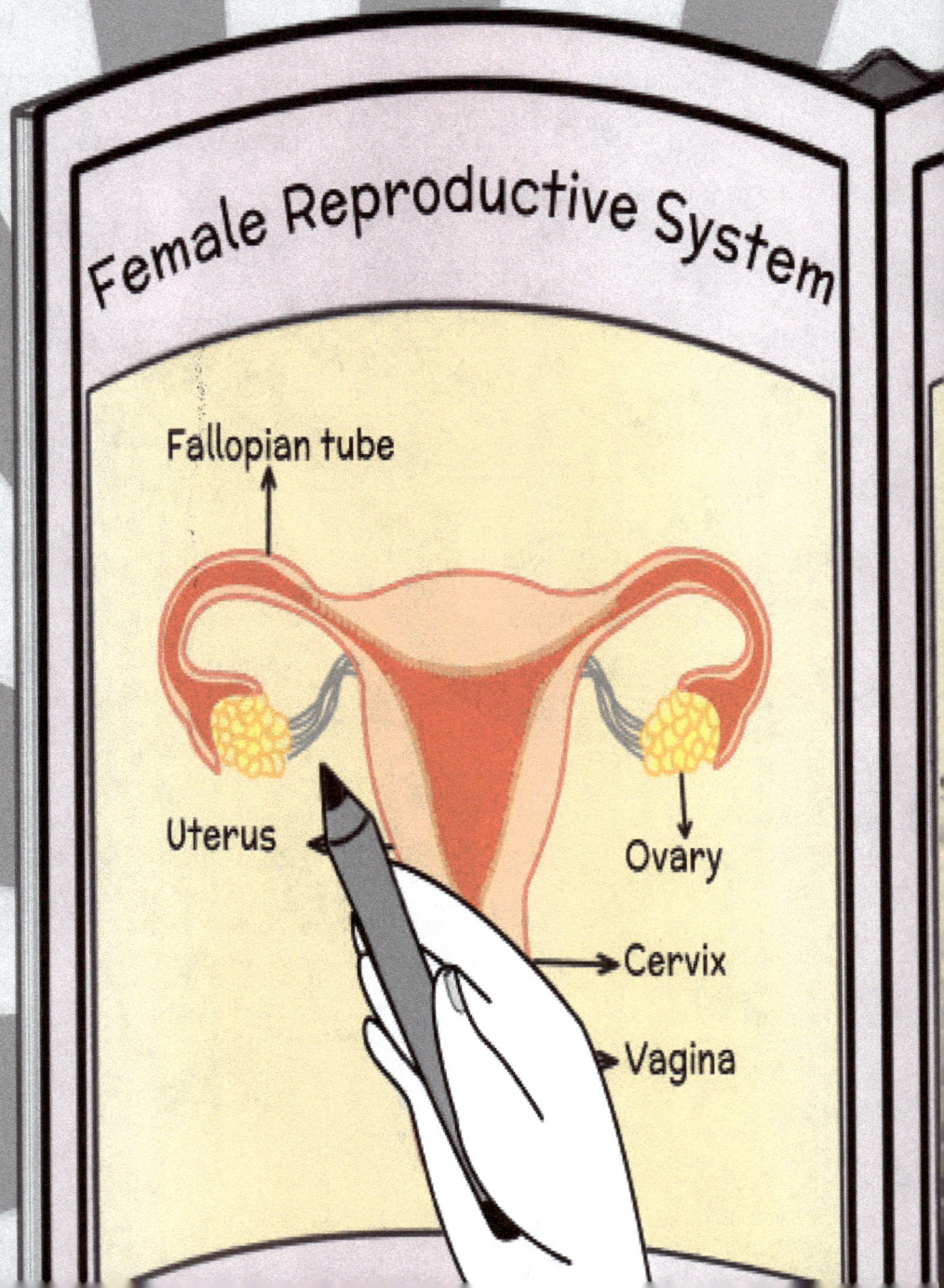

Female Reproductive System

Fallopian tube

Uterus

Ovary

Cervix

Vagina

"If the egg does not become a baby, the uterus sheds the protective walls and the lining leaves the body through the vagina."

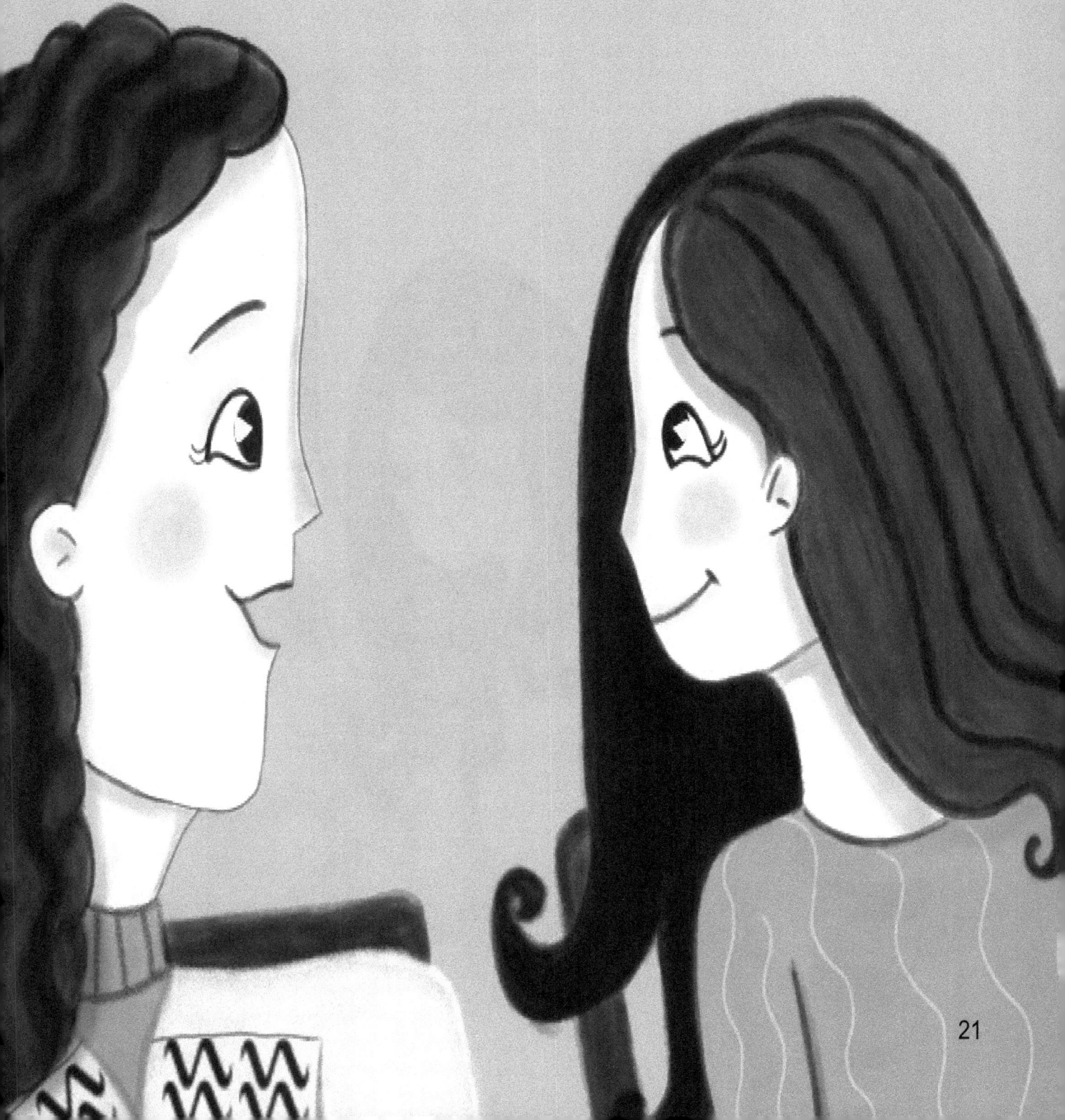

I looked at down at the book in Mamas lap watching her fingers move across the page.

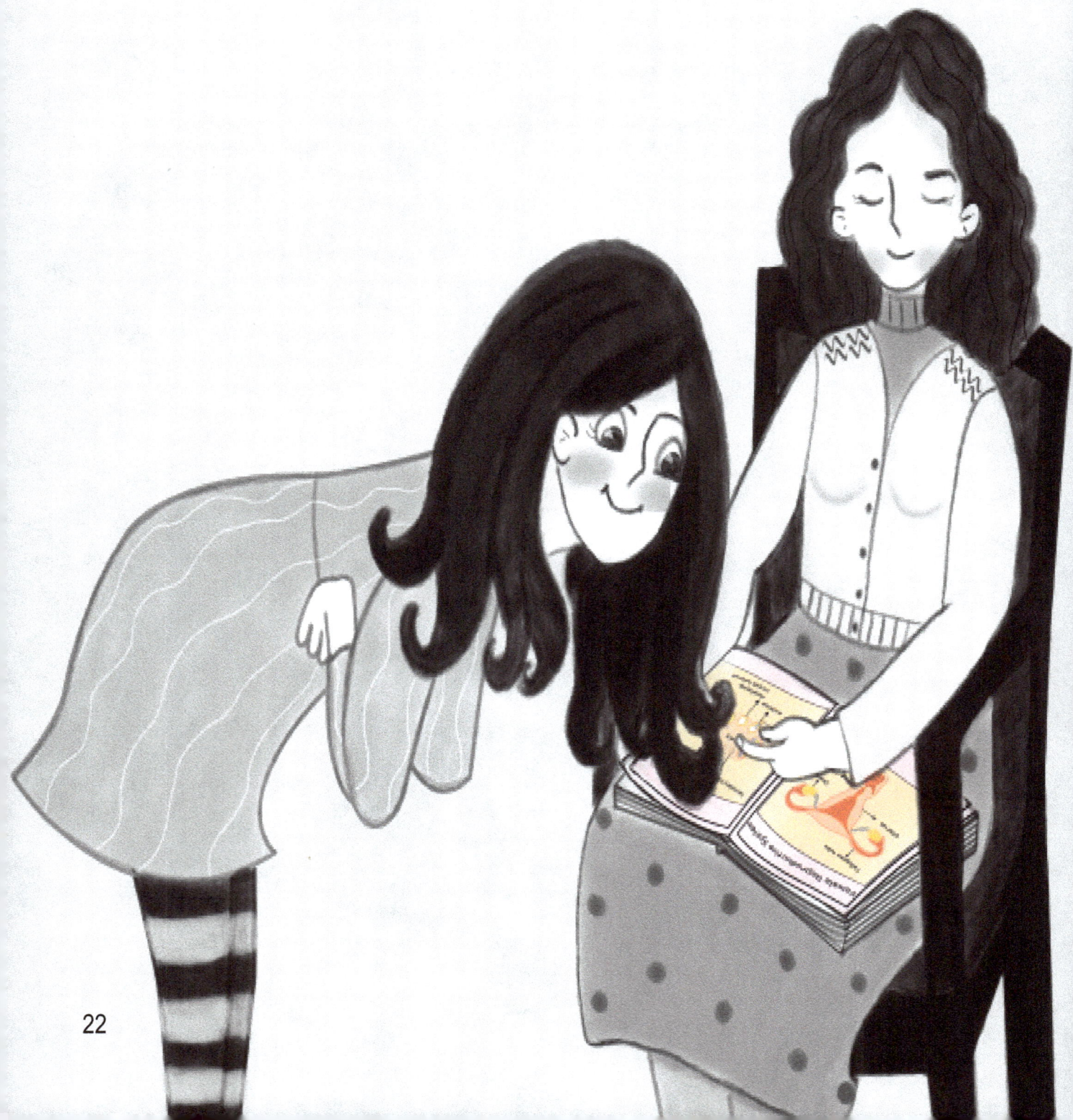

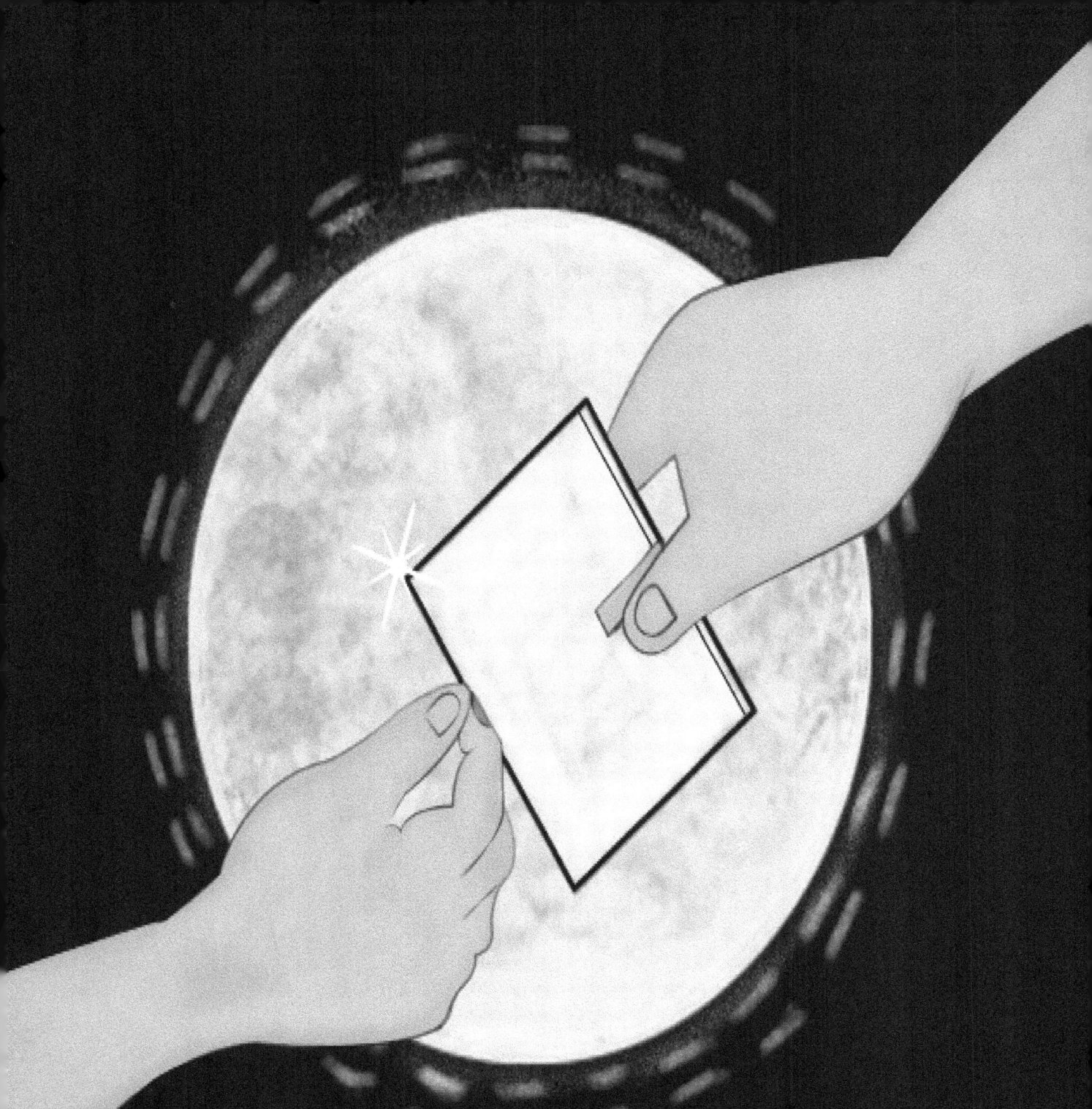

"This "flow" of fluid is what we call our "period" or "monthly" or "cycle". This is why we have sanitary pads and tampons, to collect the blood and lining that comes out of our bodies."

"It looks like a lot of blood, but really we only loose a few teaspoons of blood. The rest is the protective wall from the uterus and tissue our body doesn't need anymore". Mama closed the book and left it on the table for me to read again.

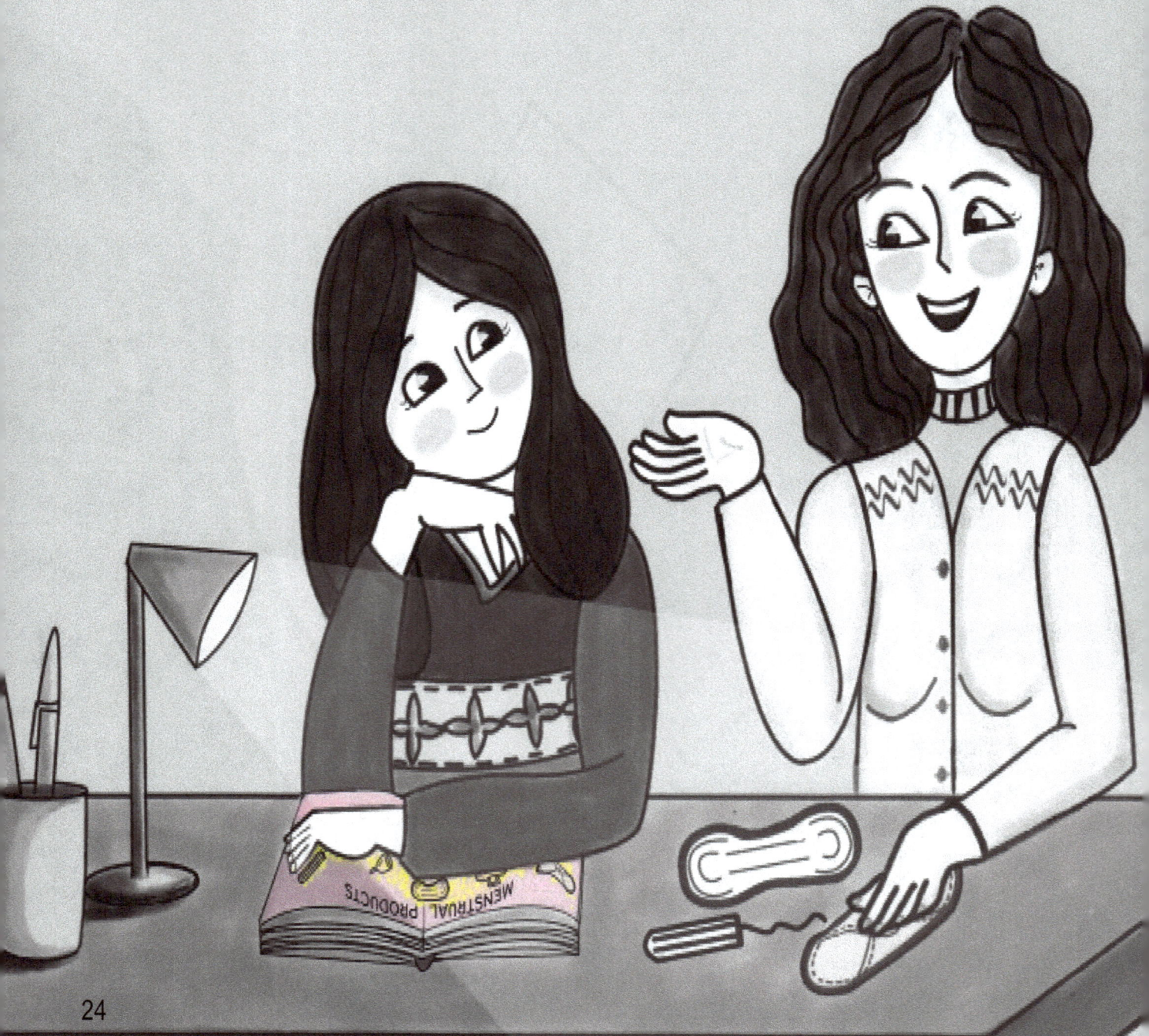

Smiling, we stood up together to look at the moon.
"Like the moon, this cycle of phases happens once a month until your body stops releasing eggs and we move into a new phase of life."

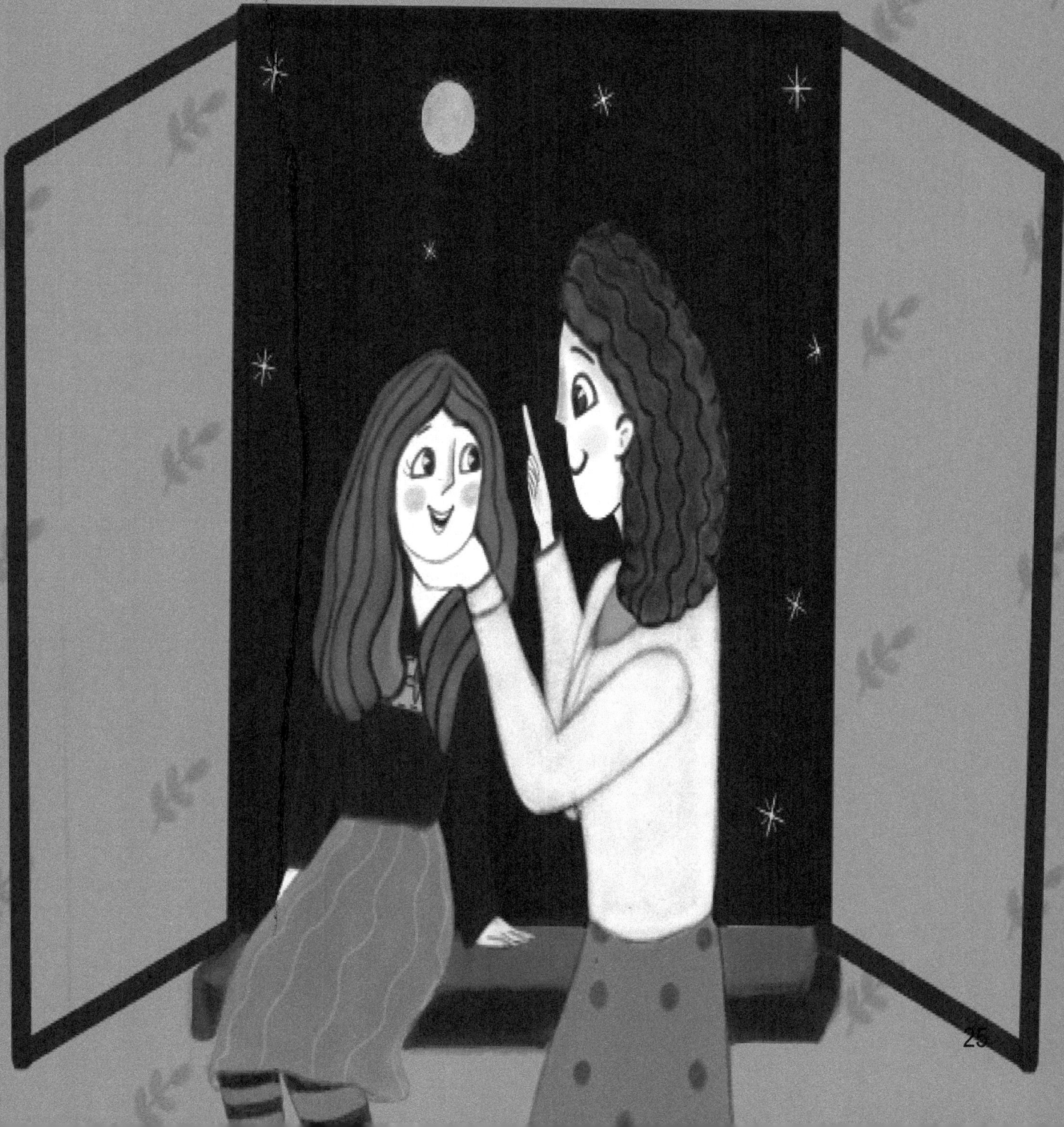

It was a lot to understand but I felt better after Mama explained why the moon visits girls and why we have Moonboxes. As we stood together watching the moon slowly rise, I was grateful for Mama.

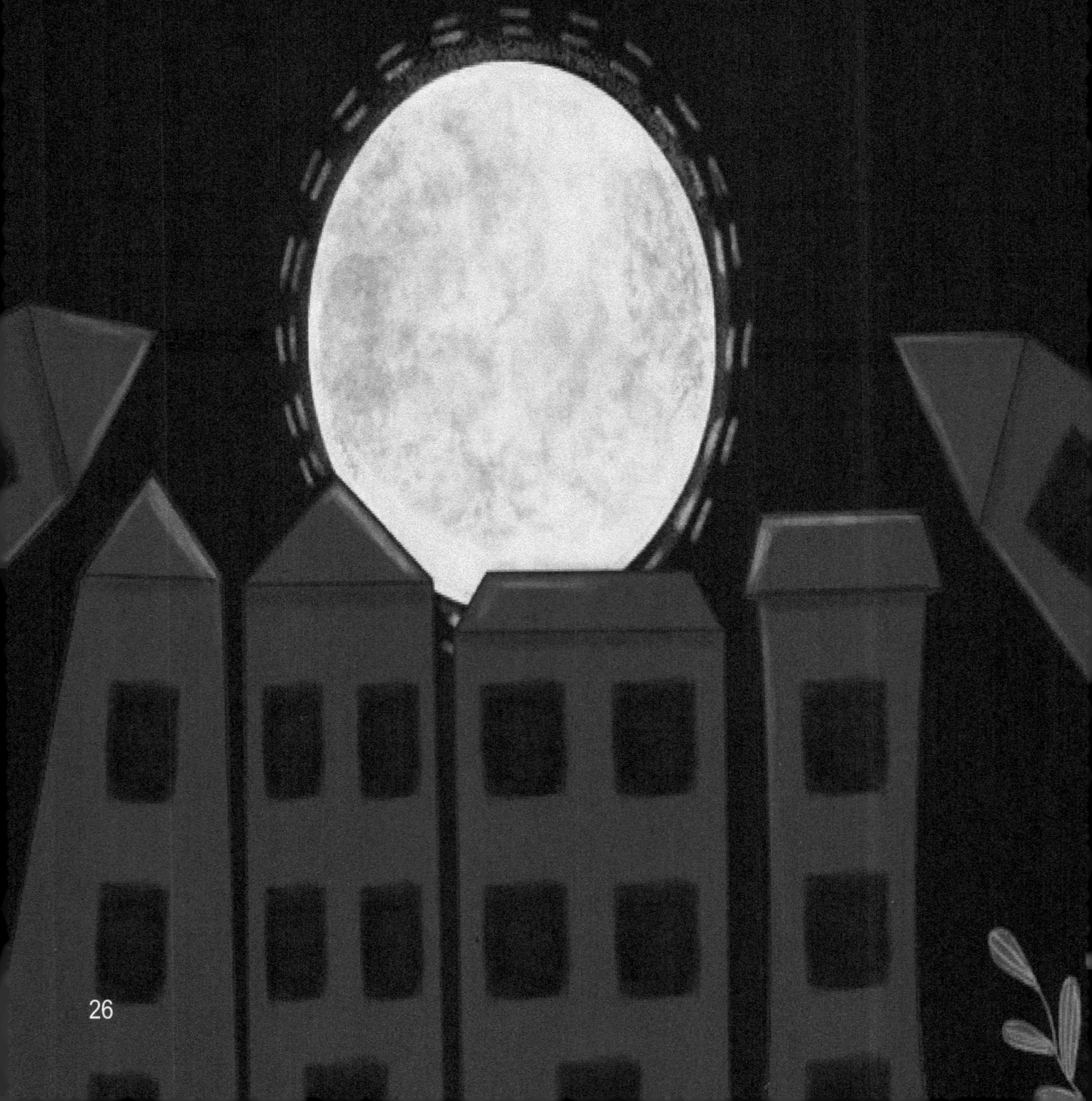

One night while I slept, the moon visited me too. When I woke up, there was blood on my bed and in my underwear! I felt embarrassed and excited and frightened.

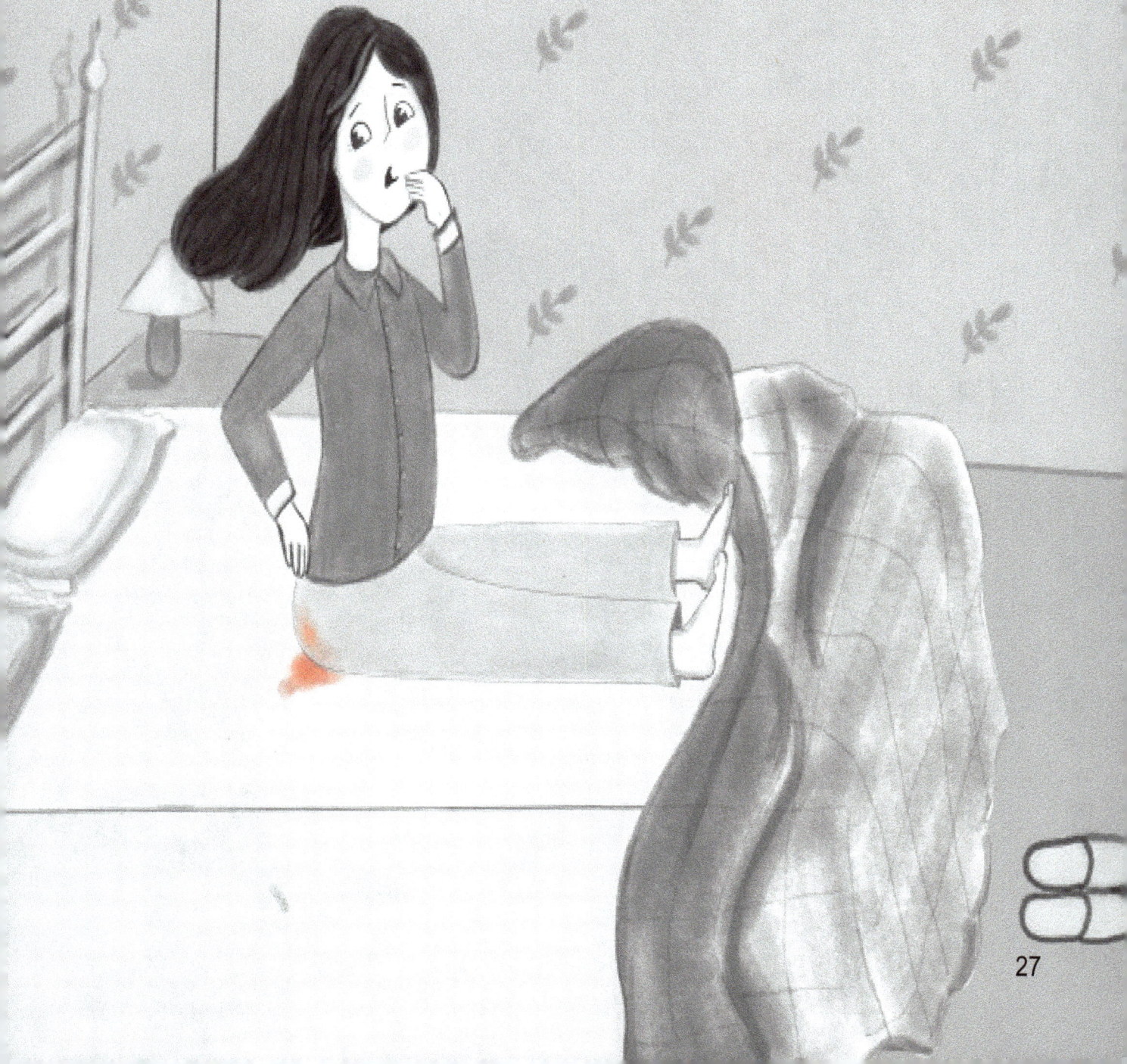

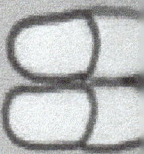

I knew
Mama would know
what to do...

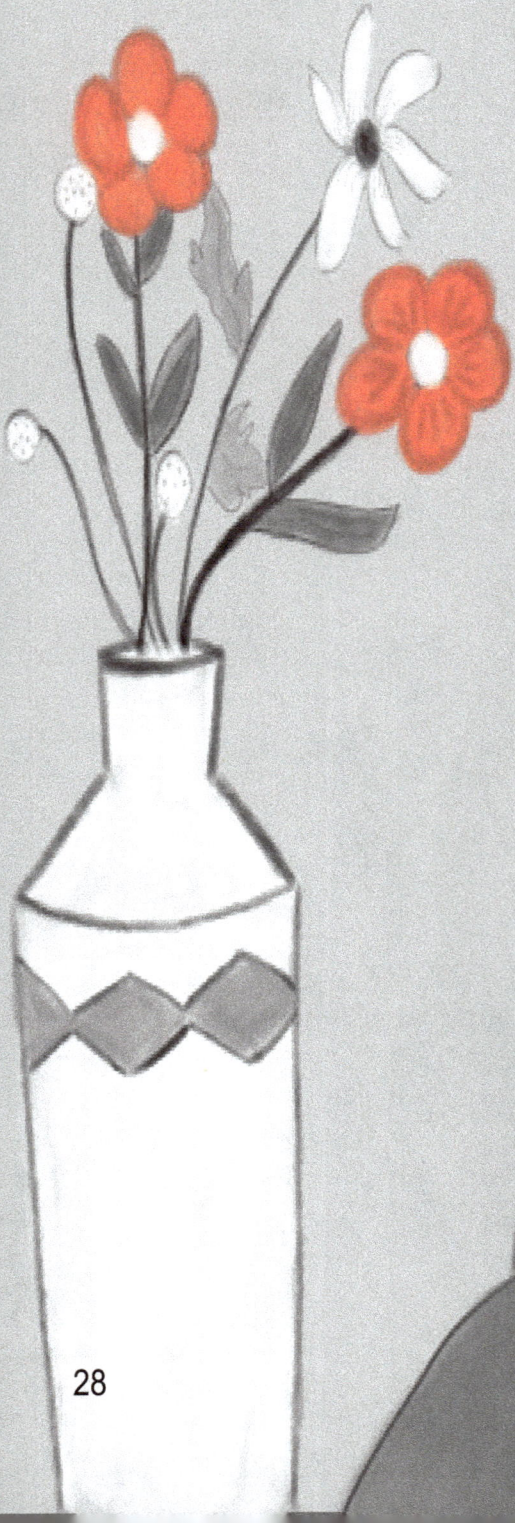

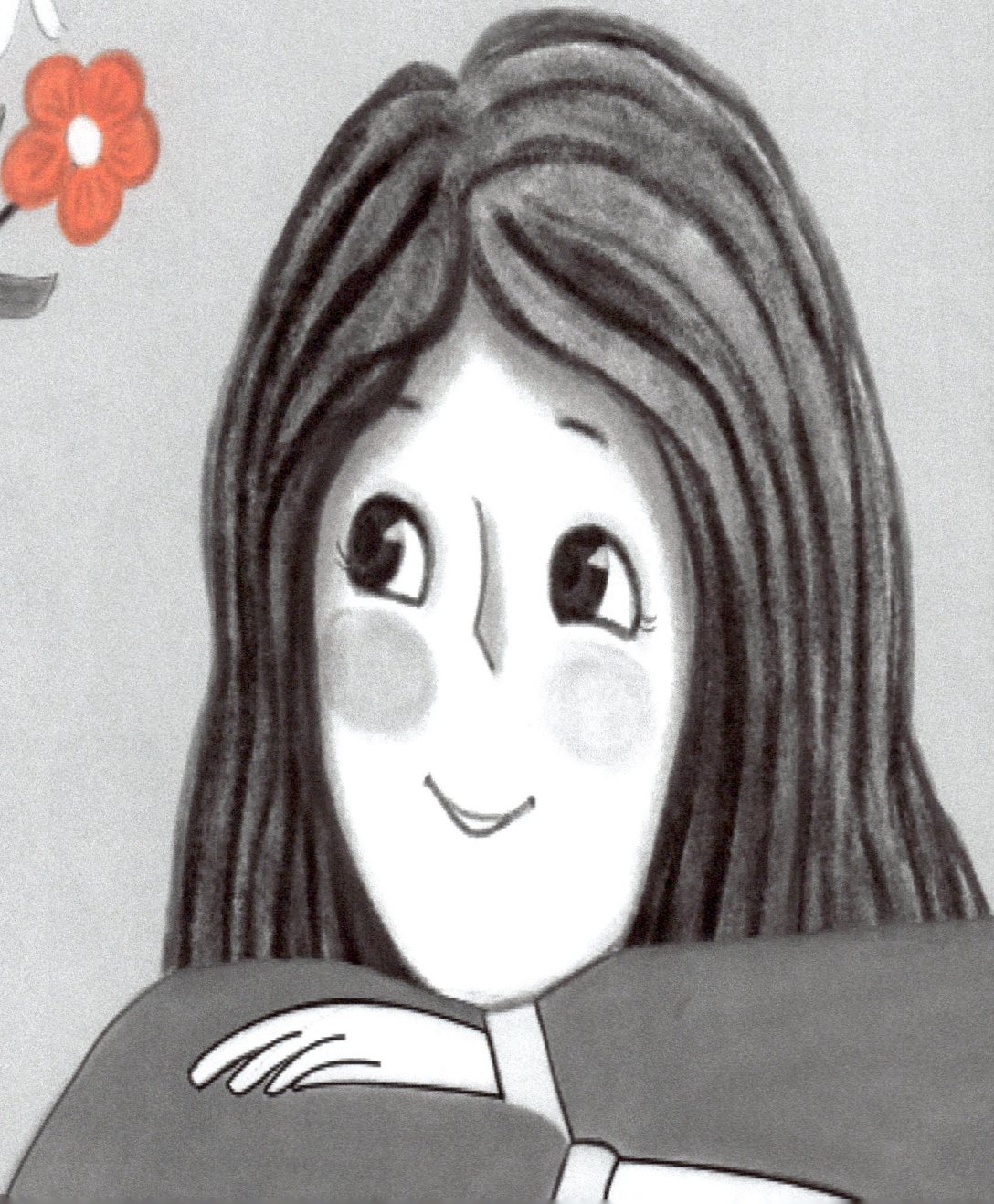

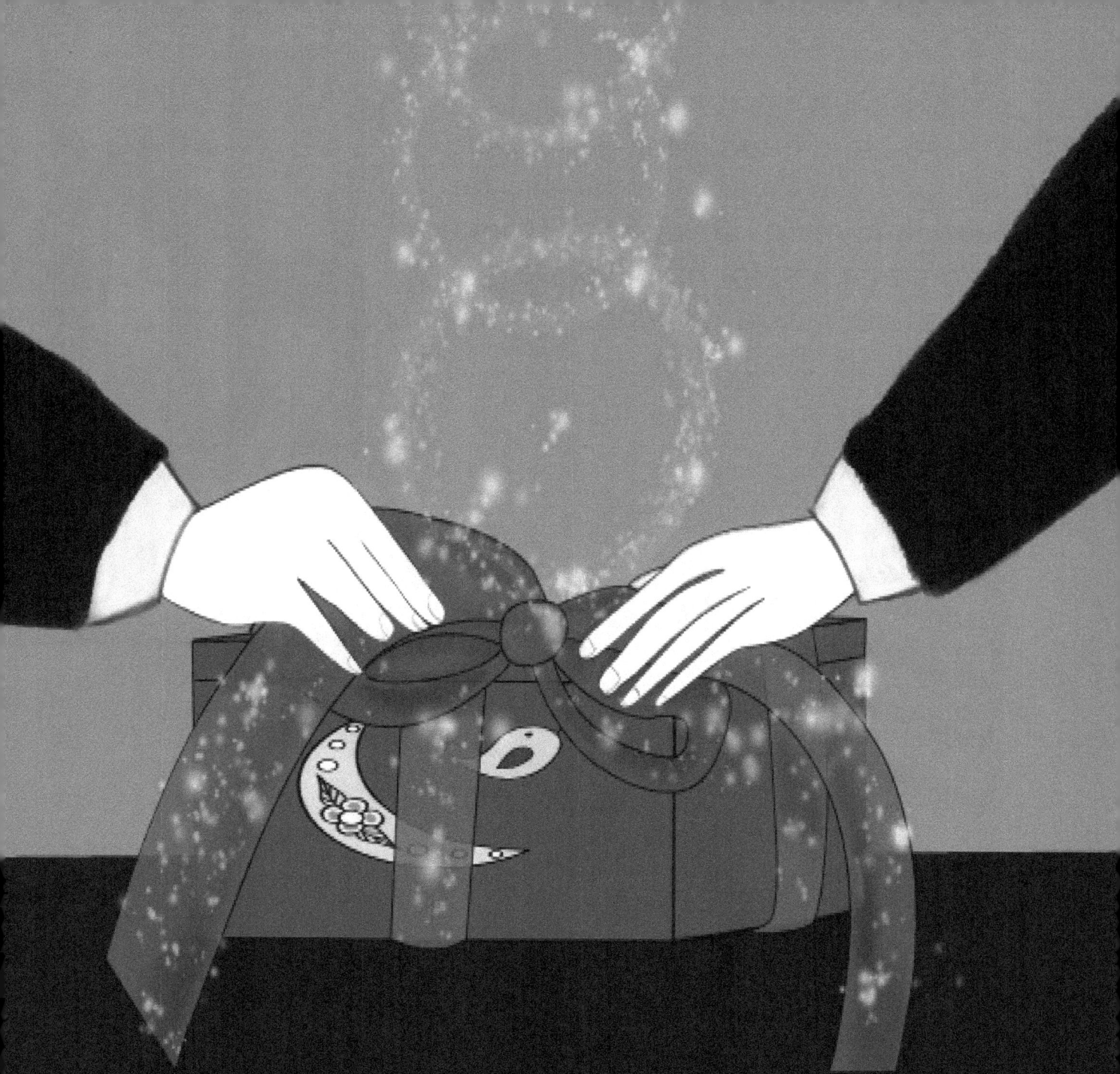

Mama handed me my very own Moonbox. The box was wrapped in a ribbon the color of moonlight. I took the box and slowly pulled on the bow.

I already knew what was inside because I had heard Mama's sewing machine while I was supposed to be asleep in my bed. It was the Moonbox Mama made just for me. Sorted by size and color. On top was what Mama knew I would liked most.

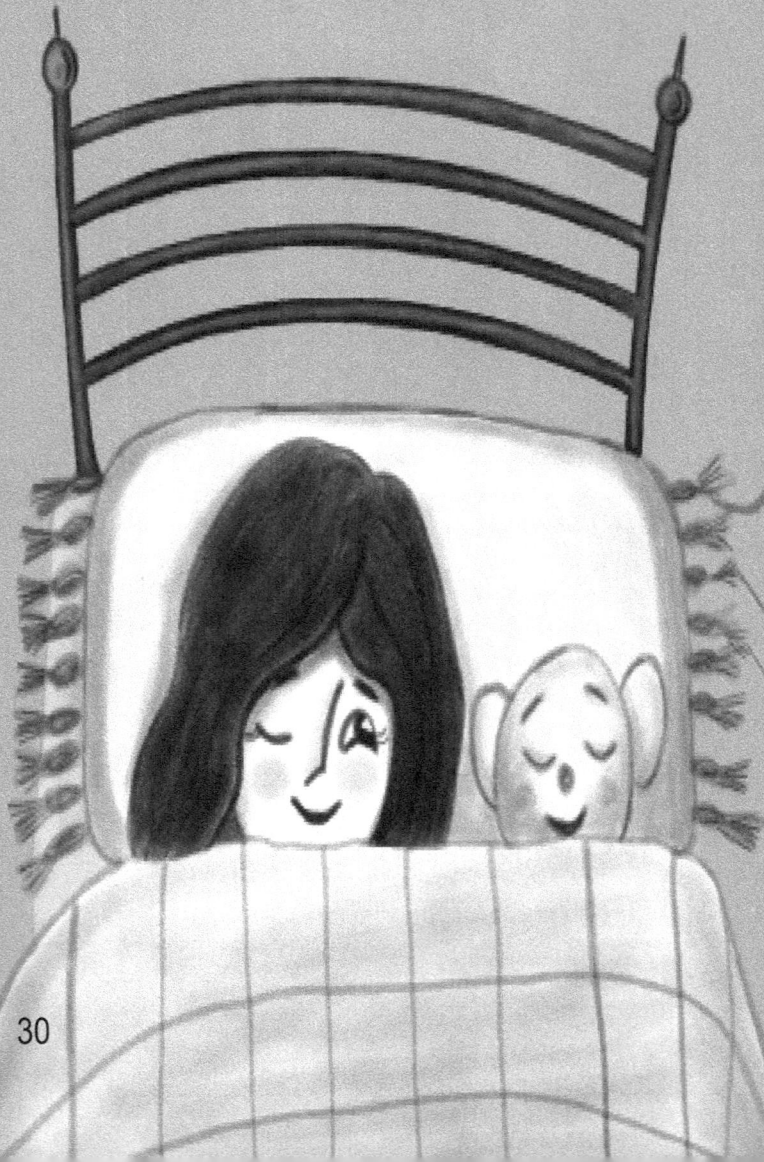

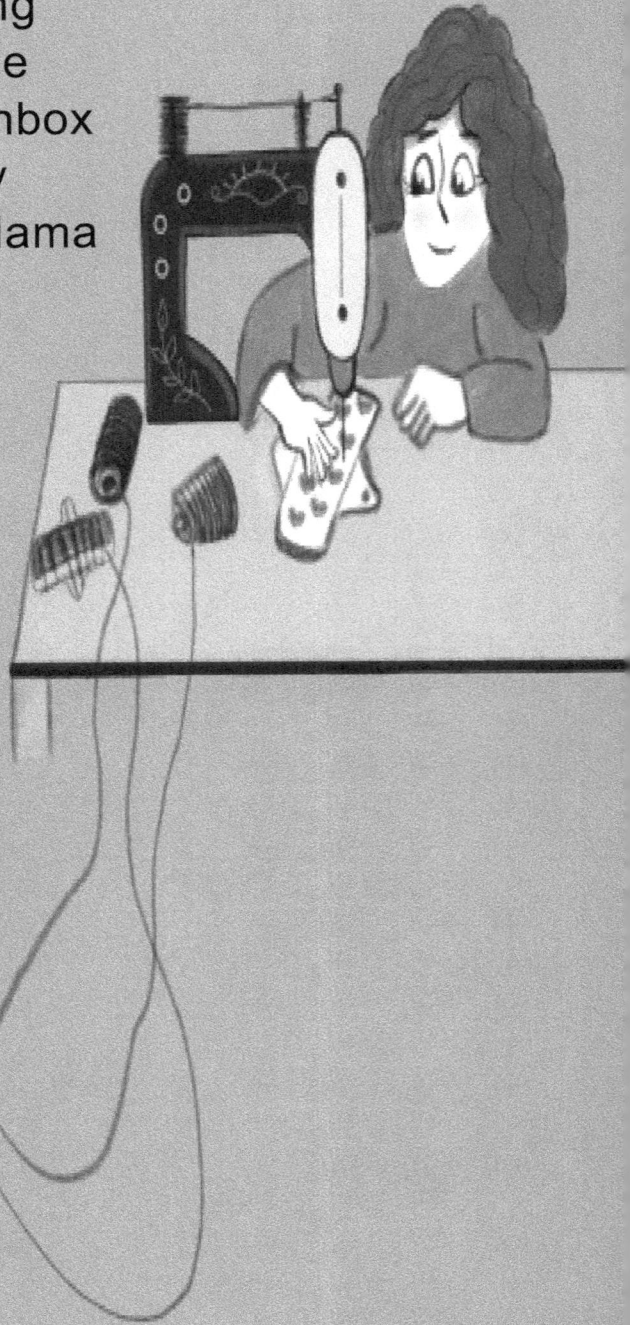

Now Mama and I share the phases of the moon in a whole new way. Mama was right, with each new moon we have a chance to make something special!

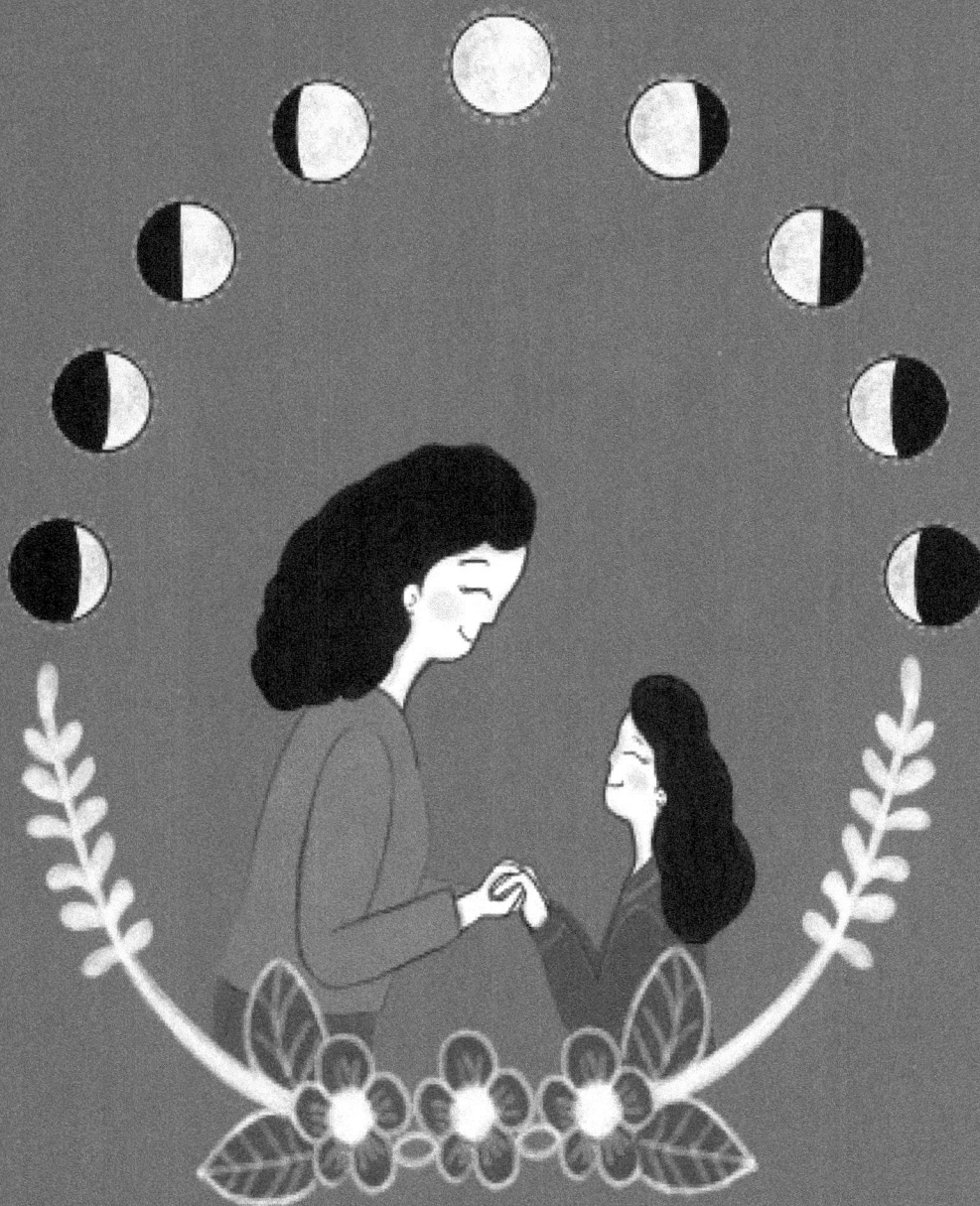

I can be anything I want to be, I just can't stop reaching for the moon!

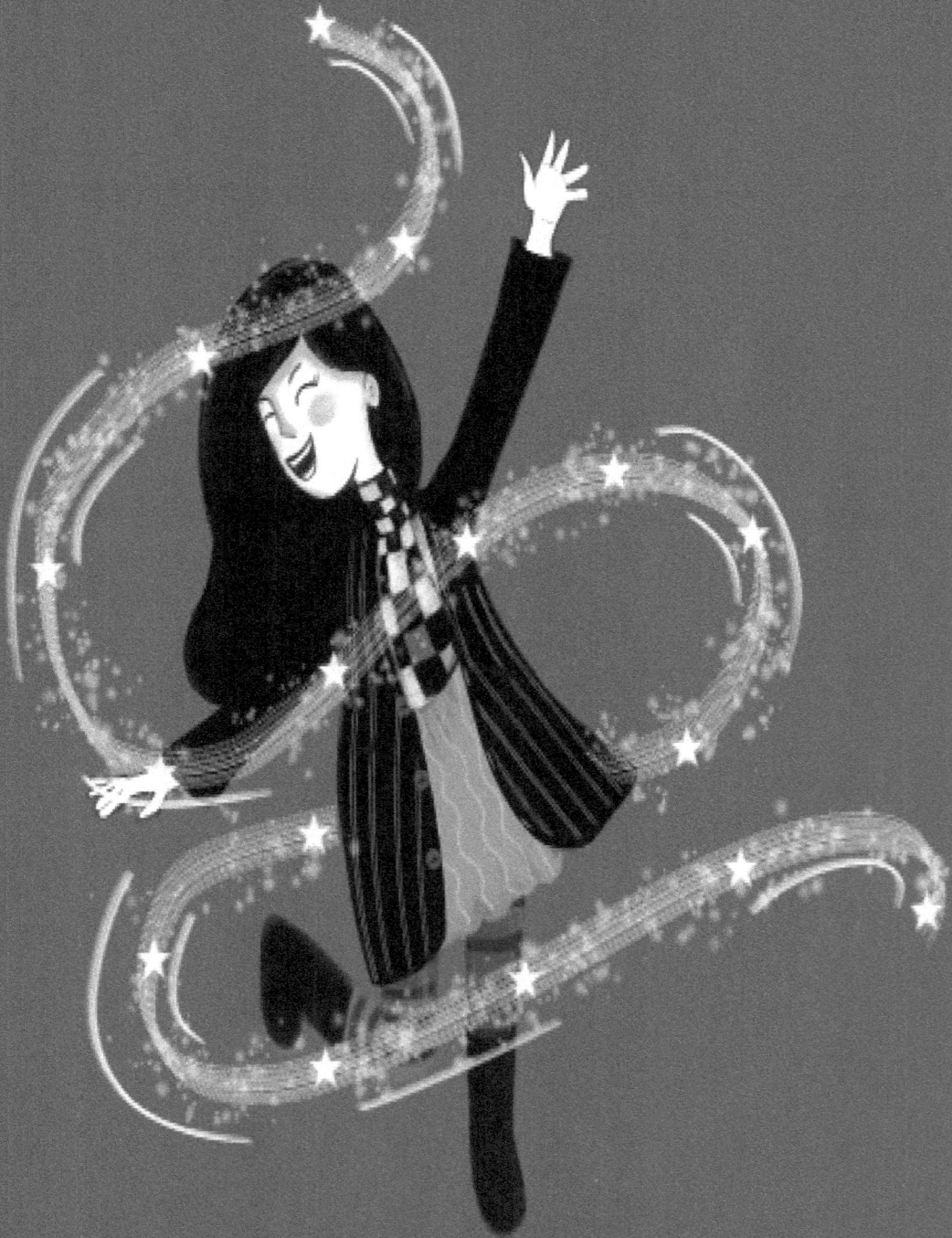

About the Author

Liz Carruth is an US Air Force veteran and has spent many years traveling the world. Liz has settled down in the Upper Peninsula of Michigan with her husband and three children. Liz loves to read books on adventure, fantasy, and history. Liz loves to write, teach, and share her knowledge with others.

About the Illustrator

Vrushali Sarwate has 15 years experience as a professional freelance illustrator and painter. She illustrates in Traditional & Digital media. Her artwork expresses a range of emotions and brings to life the imagination and thoughts of writers.

Her creative artwork has been published in children's books in English, Marathi, and Tamil languages. She has exhibited her paintings in India's art galleries. Vrushali conducts art classes and workshops for children. She learned fine art from Chitari Acadamy of Fine Art in Pune, India.

Vrushali is a gold medalist and holds a Masters in Geography and a rank topper P.G. Diploma in Environmental Management. Currently, she lives in Hong Kong with her husband and a son.

Parent Guide

How to use this book

This book is a tool to openly discuss menstruation (menses) with your child. Open discussion allows your child to ask questions in a manner that they normally wouldn't ask. This book is not a replacement for information from your own experience, knowledge, or professional medical opinions. Preparing your child about what to expect, before menstruation happens, is the best comfort and support you can provide during this exciting and scary transformation into womanhood.

Talking to your child

Discussions that make you feel awkward is often the perfect way to bond with your child! Try not to make your conversation uncomfortable for you or her. Just allow the topic to become a natural part of the conversation. Listen to your child and look for opportunities to talk to her. Keep this book handy to use as a quick reference.

Answering questions

Always speak with your child's doctor if you have any questions regarding your child's development. Like all children, not all girls will menstruate at the same time or in the same way. Some girls start younger than 8 years old and others start after age 13. One girl may have light periods and another may be a heavy bleeder. Nomatter which age your child starts menstruating, the most important step is for her to get the information regarding her body from you. You are your child's first line of communication. Just remember to *relax* and let the conversation happen naturally. Be open and honest. If you don't know how to answer her question, research her question together so you both can learn. Show her your interest in the changes that are happening to her (and her body) and chances are that she will be excited too! Menstruation should be a time of excitement and anticipation, not a lesson in monthly disappointment for years to come.

More information about menstruation

Just as our moon waxes and wanes every 28 days, the cycle of female reproduction also occurs approximately every 28 days. Which is why this monthly phenomenon goes by so many names: monthly, cycle, time of the month, "Moon Time", "Monthly friend", ect. Once menstruation ends for the first time, the cycle returns again, roughly 28 days later. Girls typically have their first period around the age of 12. Around this time, you may also notice hair growth under the arms and breast buds. If your child has not started to menstruate before 15 years of age, it is recommended you see your physician.

The Menstrual Cycle

Once a female reaches sexual maturity her body will begin to ovulate. **Ovulation** is when the ovaries release a mature egg (ovulation occurs about 14 days after her last period). The egg then travels down the fallopian tube where it can be fertilized. The **fallopian tube** is a "one way" tube (connection) from ovary to uterus. It is during ovulation that a woman is most fertile to conceive a child. Fertilization happens when a man and a woman have sexual intercourse and the man's sperm and woman's egg join together. If the egg does not get fertilized (or if the woman is not sexually active) the woman will undergo menstruation. **Menstruation** is when the uterus sheds the protective walls (endometrium) it has developed in preparation to grow and nourish a fetus (baby). The menstrual flow is made up of endometrium lining, blood, and vaginal mucus. This flow of fluid then passes through the birth canal and out of the vagina where it is collected with sanitary products. To learn more about sanitary products, refer to "**Her Options**" on page 48.

Most women will menstruate every 28 days. Some menstruate as often as every 21 days or go as long as every 45 days. As long as your child is not sexually active there should be no cause for alarm if her monthly period falls somewhere between 21-45 days. Also, the amount of fluid passed varies between women. Some women are heavy bleeders, and likewise, some are light bleeders. The average length of time bleeding should be 4-5 days with the first few days being the heaviest in flow. Although it can be alarming, if you see or feel like your child is losing a lot of blood, rest assured that the blood lost over the next few days will be quite minimal. The average menstruating woman loses approximately 6-8 teaspoons of blood during each menstruation cycle.

Advice and Guidelines for Menstruating Girls

Menstruating girls should be changing their pad or tampon every 3-4 hours. You should monitor your child's flow as heavy bleeding can take its toll on her development and cause anemia. **Anemia** is an iron deficiency caused by lack of red blood cells. When your child is menstruating, it is easy to experience low blood iron causing your child to feel depleted and fatigued. You can help your child by administering a daily vitamin that contains iron or increasing her amount of iron rich foods such as dark leafy greens to help boost iron levels. If you are concerned that your child might be experiencing anemia or experiencing heavy periods, contact your child's doctor.

Heavy periods are defined by the Center for Disease Control as:
- Needing to change your pad or tampon after less than 2 hours
- Needing to double up on pads to control menstrual flow
- Passing clots larger than a quarter (1 inch or 25mm)
- Menstrual flow that keeps one from doing normal activities
- Menstruation longer than 7 days in a row
- Pain in your stomach and shortness of breath

Cysts/fibroids/polyps

Cysts, fibroids, & polyps are all different kinds of growths that can develop inside the female reproductive organs. These growths are typically non-cancerous. Although it is uncommon for younger menstruating girls to have growths or cysts, these unusual developments can cause major discomfort, especially if a cyst bursts. Learn the signs and symptoms of potential growths and cysts so you can help your child receive medical care and treatment.

The symptoms of cysts, fibroids, and polyps are:

- Lower abdominal pain or pelvic pressure
- Sudden and severe sharp pain if an ovarian cyst burst
- Nausea or vomiting along with pain in the abdomen
- Heavy or prolonged menstrual bleeding
- Pelvic pain or very painful menstruation
- Vaginal bleeding after physical activity

Caring for your Menstruating Girl

Eating chocolates & watching RomComs is not an appropriate level of care for a newly menstruating girl. A healthy diet and moderate exercise are going to be her best defense against menstrual fatigue and cramps. Fruits and vegetables rich in iron will help her maintain iron levels and energy while menstruating. Examples of iron rich foods: dark green leafy vegetables, fortified cereals, dried fruit, black beans, eggs, ect.

Exercise should not be overlooked while menstruating. Women assume exercise is going to make cramps and fatigue worse but there is some research that shows exercise can help relieve menstruation symptoms. If your child is feeling up to light exercise, such as walking or jogging, encourage her to continue with a regular exercise routine.

Puberty is the driving force behind the transition from adolescent to adult. As with any change, there may also be emotional adjustments that need to be addressed. You may find your child to be increasingly disagreeable or easily upset, saddened, or angry. Although these changes might seem "out of the blue" or "not her usual self", they are completely normal. The term "moody teenager" has been used for a long time, and for good reason. Mood changes associated with menstruation have their own medical term: PreMenstrual Syndrome or **PMS**. **PMS** is characterized by "moodiness" approximately 4 days before her period and ends shortly after her menstrual fluid starts to flow.

PMS symptoms include:
- **Mood Swings**- a rapid change in emotions such as happiness to anger, sadness, or uncontrollable laughter. Mood swings might be anything "out of the norm" for your child's typical demeanor. Mood swings can also be characterized by crankiness, sadness, whining, irritability, and anxiety.

- **Tiredness**- your child is bound to be exhausted during and after her period. Afterall, her body is working hard to keep her in a constant state of preparation for pregnancy, but don't worry! As long as your child is not sexually active, there is no need to be concerned because her body is doing *exactly* what it is supposed to be doing. Give her the time she needs to rest up and relax.
- **Food Cravings**- she may have the desire to eat rich foods such as sweets, meats, chips, and/or "junk foods" to replenish the vitamins and minerals her body is consuming. Instead of foods that are high in sugar and of little or no nutritional value, encourage her to make smart food choices that will replenish her body, not just fill her with empty calories which can lead to a poor body image, undesirable weight gain, and emotional challenges.
- **Skin Changes**- acne and oily skin are some of the changes you will notice with your child. Explain how good hygiene and a nutrient-rich diet will help combat oily skin and acne. To learn more about hygiene for your child, refer to "**Her Hygiene**" on page 62.
- **Physical Discomforts**- just before the start and during menstruation girls can experience physical discomforts. These discomforts include bloating, backaches, sore breasts, lower abdomen cramps, headaches, constipation, or diarrhea.

Relieving your Child's Discomfort

Discomfort is to be expected while your child menstruates. Cramps are common as the uterus is contracting to shed the endometrium lining. These cramps can range from mild discomfort, to very painful and can disrupt daily life.

Things a caretaker can do to ease these discomforts:
- Heating pad or hot water bottle over the lower abdomen to help relieve cramps
- Oral, over the counter, medications such as Tylenol®, Motrin®, or Midol® can be administer to your child to relieve the pain and cramps associated with menstruation
- Ensure your menstruating child is getting adequate sleep
- Drinking Water
- Daily vitamin
- Stress management
- Communication, empathy, support, and understanding

Sanitary options

There are *many* options these days when it comes to managing menstrual flow. It can seem overwhelming to a caretaker when they are not familiar with these options. "**Her Options**" section of this book covers nearly all known sanitary products in thorough detail. The most common way menstrual fluid is collected are pads and tampons. In many cultures there exists a silent stigma that women should be embarrassed to be seen buying pads and tampons, let alone *talk* about their period. This stigma can end with your help. Let purchasing pads and tampons become a fun experience. Use this time to connect with your child about how nice it is to be able to communicate and provide for her needs. If you are unfamiliar with menstrual options please refer to "**Her Options**" section on page 48 and learn with your child about what she can use to make her menstrual cycle most comfortable and manageable.

NOTE: Commercial (disposable) sanitary products can contain chemicals, synthetic materials, and fragrances that can cause rashes and/or irritation to the delicate skin and pH levels of the vagina. Scientific evidence regarding exposure to these chemicals and the synthetic materials found in some of these menstrual products, such as Dioxin, can lead to reproductive diseases and cancer. Become an informed consumer about disposable menstrual products and how they impact your child's reproductive health, as well as our environment. Consider using reusable options such as cloth pads, menstrual cups/discs, and period panties to combat pollution and reduce your child's exposure to potentially harmful chemicals and synthetic materials commonly found in many commercial, disposable sanitary products.

An Important Note for Parents/Guardians

There are plenty of myths surrounding the use of tampons and virginity. Although it is a parent/guardian's choice to allow your child to use tampons, you can rest assured it is completely safe for your child to use a tampon without damaging the hymen and her virginity. The following quotes were used with permission from Proctor and Gamble and Tampax® regarding tampons and virginity:

> "First things first, your hymen doesn't actually "break" — it stretches. While it's possible that a tampon will stretch your hymen, it's also possible that your hymen has stretched in other ways already, or will, or won't stretch even when you do have sex. Tampons are small, and can usually be inserted through the existing opening of your hymen (how do you think all the blood and blood clots on your period come out?) Sometimes even first-time penetrative sex doesn't even stretch the hymen all the way or as much as you think it would."
> Source: https://tampax.com/en-us/tampon-truths/do-tampons-take-your-virginity/

What you *do* need to be concerned and attentive regarding tampons is Toxic Shock Syndrome (TSS). **Toxic Shock Syndrome** is an infection caused by Staphylococcus (Staph) bacteria. There has been a lot of concern that tampons are the only way to get TSS but that simply isn't true. The tampon is a medical device and made under sterile conditions. *Hygiene* is the cause of the TSS infection. Also used with permission from Proctor and Gamble and Tampax® :

"You can get it (TSS) while using pads or menstrual cups, or no period protection at all. Anyone can get TSS. Even men and children can get TSS, and only about half of TSS infections are related to menstruation. Some other ways people develop TSS include insect bites, skin infections, or surgery."

Hygiene is the best defense against TSS. Inform your child about how to keep herself clean while using tampons and during her menstruation. Talk with her about your concerns and the risks associated with using tampons. Tampons are a great tool to keep your child from missing out on everyday fun and public activities. To find out more, check out www.tampax.com online or talk to your child's doctor about how to use a tampon safely.

Congratulations for taking this important step in guiding your child through menstruation!

Girls Guide

Starting menstruation can be an exciting and frightening experience, but with the right tools and information it doesn't have to be scary! That's why this book's section was created with *you* in mind. Sometimes there are things you might want to know but are unsure how to ask or are too embarrassed to ask. That's OK!! Just remember: talking about your feelings and experiences (communication) during this time is one of the most important skills you will have as you grow older! If you are unable to find the answers to your questions it's important to ask/talk to a parent, guardian, or trusted adult such as a teacher, aunt, or doctor.

Your Body

Your body is an amazing creation! Your body is the vessel that propels your thoughts into actions, such as giving your friend a high-five or dancing to the beat of your favorite song. Some actions and changes are made on their own, like your body transitioning from a child to an adult. This change is called puberty. **Puberty** is the process by which your body makes *physical* changes from a child's body into an adult, such as growing breasts and the start of menstruation. The driving force behind these changes are hormones. **Hormones** are the invisible chemicals inside our body that tell parts of our body how to work. By the end of puberty, an adult woman is able to sexually reproduce. Women are born with sexual organs, both inside and outside of her body. These organs are needed to be able to reproduce.

External Reproductive Organs

- **Breasts** (boobs) are the fatty round tissues on the front of a woman's chest. These fatty tissues hold the milk glands that will produce milk after birth to feed your baby. Around the time of your first menstruation, your breasts will begin to develop. They will continue to grow as your body matures into an adult.
- **Genitals** (external sex organs) is a word that describes the external parts of the reproductive system. The official name for a woman's external reproductive organ is the **Vulva**.
- The vulva has 3 major parts:
  - **Labia**-(lips of the vagina) the folds of skin on each side of the vulva
  - **Urethra**-the narrow opening above the vaginal opening used to urinate
  - **Vaginal opening**- is the passageway to the internal reproductive organs; it is the larger opening of the vulva and the opening for menstrual fluid to comes out

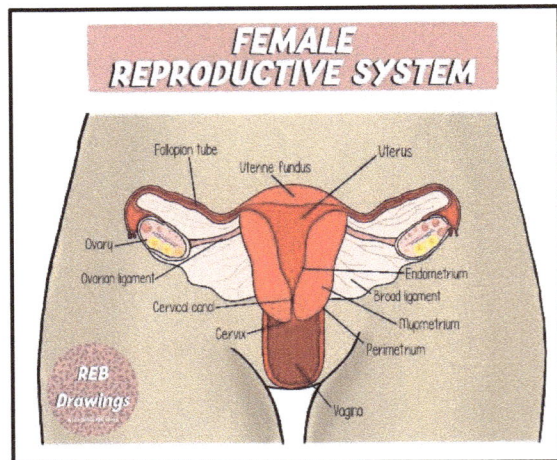

Illustration by: REB Drawings
Used with permission from REB Drawings

Internal Reproductive Organs

- ○ **Ovaries**-the bean shaped organs that release the egg needed for reproduction; women have 2 ovaries.
- ○ **Fallopian tube**-the narrow tube connecting the ovary to the uterus; serves as the pathway for the egg to enter the uterus
- ○ **Uterus**-(womb) the "pear shaped" organ where a baby develops; the inner lining of the uterus is the **endometrium**. The endometrium is what comes out of the vagina during menstruation.
- ○ **Cervix**-the narrow organ separating the uterus from the vagina. It is like the "gateway" to the uterus or vagina.
- ○ **Vagina**-(birth canal) is the long muscular opening that connects the cervix and vagina. This is the opening where menstrual fluid comes out of the body.

What *is* Menstruation?

Menstruation is a process (or cycle) your body goes through each month. Every 28 days to be exact! As you grow older, your body is doing amazing things such as practicing to grow a baby inside you. Every 28 days your body grows a special layer or lining inside your **uterus** (your body's organ that holds a growing and developing baby). Around 14 days after your last period, an egg is released from one of your 2 ovaries. The egg flows down your fallopian tube and into the uterus. The egg only has a few days to live and wait to be fertilized. If the egg is not fertilized, the egg dissolves and is reabsorbed back into your body. When the egg begins to dissolve the special lining inside your uterus (called the endometrium) breaks down. This lining, along with mucus and blood, mix together and flow out of your body through the **vagina** (your private). Without the use of something to collect these fluids, women would constantly battle blood stains, odors, and illnesses from an unsanitary mess. This is why women use sanitary products: to collect the flow of fluid that comes out of your body. The process of preparing your uterus for a new egg, causes our body to discharge the old blood, mucus, and uterine tissue is what we call **menstruation** or your period.

Menstruation (or your period) goes by a lot of different names. Girls talk about their periods using euphemisms (words or expressions that are used in place of another). Girls do this so other people who might be listening won't know what you're talking about or because they are embarrassed. Nobody wants to announce to the world they are on their period! Lots of different cultures and people think your period is a topic we shouldn't talk about but that simply isn't true. Talking about sensitive topics can help others to understand how you're feeling or what you're going through. Although each of our experiences with menstruation is completely unique to each of us, we *do* need to rely on our family and friends to learn about how to care for ourselves during your period. We hear menstruation called by a lot of different names, some of these names are funny or quirky, but it's up to us to know what these sayings mean when we hear them. Here are just a few of the common euphemisms of menstruation: "Period," "Cycle," "Time of the Month," "On the Rag," "Aunt Flow," "Shark Week," My "Aunt is visiting," " Code Red," ect.

Question and Answer Time

A lot of questions come to mind when we are expecting to experience something new. Your first period is no exception. The following is a list of common questions and answers girls have about menstruation:

- **Will it hurt?**
  - Periods can be painful, especially when it's your first time. Pain with our periods is because the uterus is contracting (or squeezing) to encourage the lining to break down and flow out the body. This pain is usually called cramps. We can treat our cramps with rest, using a heating-pad over the abdomen, and medicine such as Tylenol®, Motrin®, or Midol®. If your cramps get bad enough, let an adult know and they can make sure you get the recommended dose of medication. You may also experience sore and tender areas near the brown spots or nipples on your chest. This is the part of the body where your breasts will begin to grow as you develop into a young woman. This happens around the time of your first menstruation.

- **Will I smell?**
  - In general, you should not smell just because you are on your period. Personal hygiene (bathing regularly) determines how bad or good a person smells. It is recommended to bathe daily while you are on your period to clean up any blood and bacteria that may collect in your groin. Because you are going to be changing your sanitary products every 3-4 hours there shouldn't be too much a concern about smelling bad. Period blood does have a distinct blood scent; kind of like "iron" or "metal". That's because our blood has a lot of iron in it! The smell you notice should be faint and since you should be bathing daily and changing your sanitary products regularly the smell should be minimal.

- **Can I still swim and play sports?**
  - Of course! It is recommended to exercise while on your period as it is said to help keep the worst of the cramps at bay. There are lots of sanitary products a girl can choose from and some of these products are designed for sports and swimming. Tampons or menstrual cups are a good choice as these products are worn inside the vagina to collect menstrual fluid. Period panties or a heavy and extra-long pad can provide that extra layer of protection a girl needs when worried about breakthrough bleeding. So YES! Continue to do the things you love, never let your period hold you back from enjoying life.

- **How do I tell my parents/guardians when I start my period?**
  - Open and honest communication is the best way to connect with family and friends. Starting your period means you're becoming a woman but that doesn't mean you are one yet. You will still need a parent or guardian to provide the sanitary products you will be needing. If you are not comfortable telling them yourself then you can tell a trusted teacher, aunt/uncle, or friend who can inform your parents or guardian that you have started. This should not be anything to worry or stress about because we

all go through it! Just remember your family loves and cares about you and will be proud of what you are able to accomplish.

- **Will my friends get a period?**
  - Yep chances are pretty close to 100% that all your female friends will get their period too. All of our bodies grow at different rates. Some girls start their periods younger than 10 and some don't start till after 15 but most of the time girls start around 12 years old. Around this time, you may notice a different type of course, dark, thick hair under your arms, legs, and on the exterior of your vagina called the **Vulva**. This hair is called **pubic hair** or body hair. Your breasts (boobs) will begin to grow and may begin to be sore and tender. If you're ever concerned about your body and how it's functioning, ask your parents or guardian or trusted adult and they should be able to answer your questions.

- **Will anyone make fun of me for my choice of sanitary product?**
  - Your choice in sanitary products is as unique as you are. What might work for one girl might not work for another. Each of us have differences in our bodies, some of us are tall and some are short, but all female **anatomy** (the way our body looks and functions inside) is the same. Our unique body shapes can make the way our fluids flow onto our sanitary products more or less effective. For example, some women bleed in the center or their pad while someone else might flow to the front or the back of the pad. Someone might be allergic to a product and may need to use something that most people don't use. For example, one girl might need to use a sea sponge vs a tampon because something in the tampon may cause her an allergic reaction. Each of us has the opportunity to use whatever sanitary product we like, with parent or guardian permission. Some sanitary products might make others uncomfortable such as tampons or menstrual cups/discs because they are inserted into the vagina and some people are uncomfortable with the idea of things being inside of us. Some girls choose to use cloth/homemade pads because they are earth friendly or because they have allergies to store bought products. No matter which product you use it does not make you a bad person. You can't let it bother you that someone doesn't "like' or approve of your choice. Sanitary products are *all* medical devices and are used for the same purpose: *to collect and dispose of menstrual fluid*. Just remember your period, your choice. You are in control of your flow and you do that by what makes you most comfortable. For a list of options for you to choose from check out "**Her Options**" on page 48 and decide what you want to try with a parent or guardian and start building your Moonbox!

- **Do I need to keep pads/tampons with me?**
  - Yes, you should always keep a clean/unopened sanitary product with you in your backpack or purse. Even though you expect your period every 28 days, sometimes you don't know when or where you will be when it starts so be prepared for when it does. A fresh pair of underwear is not a bad idea either because occasionally we have leaks or start and it can get onto our underwear. The internet is full of cute reusable storage bags called "wet bags" to place clean or dirty sanitary products in. If your period sneaks up and you're not prepared to start your period, you can use

rolled up toilet paper or a paper towel placed into the bottom of your underwear until you can ask an adult (such as a teacher, school nurse, or parent) for sanitary products. For more on wet bags check out "**Her Hygiene**" on page 62.

- **How often will I have a period? What happens if I miss my period?**
  - Your period should happen every 28 days or once a month. Sometimes girls start every 21 days or go as long as every 45 days. Our emotions, physical activities, and hormones can play a part in our menstrual cycle. If you are an anxious or worried person it can delay or make you miss a period. If you play very intense sports, it can delay or make you miss your period. **Hormones** are the invisible chemicals inside our body that tell parts of our body how to work. Sometimes these hormones can be out of balance and can cause our period to be delayed or missed altogether. Diet and exercise can affect your period too. Always choose to eat healthy, whole foods, and get plenty of exercise and sleep.
- **How often will I need to change my pad or tampon?**
  - Your period generally starts heavy and then gets lighter over the next few days. The general rule of thumb: change your pad or tampon every 3-4 hours (generally the first few days are the heaviest) As your period begins to slow down, you may be able to change it every 5-6 hours and eventually once a day as it begins to stop. Bleeding can last anywhere from 2-7 days. If you begin to soak through pads or tampons faster than every 2 hours you need to talk to your parents or guardian as you may be experiencing heavy periods and may need to talk to a doctor.
- **How long does it last?**
  - Periods usually last anywhere from 2-7 days.
- **What about when I sleep?**
  - When you're on your period you will bleed all night and all day until it stops. Sleeping can be worrisome if you're new to menstruation. Some good ideas to get a good night sleep are: sleep with overnight pads or heavy extra-long pads as your flow may move more as you toss and turn during the night. You can place an old towel underneath you while you sleep in case of leaks. A tampon, menstrual cup, or menstrual disc is a good option to collect your flow while you sleep. Period panties with a pad will protect you and your bed from leaking if you are concerned about leaking during the night.

Her Options

Sanitary options come in *many* forms these days from underwear with a pad embedded into it to silicone cups you wear inside your vagina to collect menstrual fluid. Some sanitary options are old as time and are still used today like the sea sponge. Some are newer takes of old concepts such as the cloth pad. Each sanitary option and device will be discussed in great detail in the following pages. To keep it simple, an "**External**" and "**Internal**" options list has been created to help you decide what you want to use inside or outside your body.

Each page will feature its **disposable** and **reusable** versions and how to use them.

Disposable: one-time use sanitary product; use once and throw it away.
Reusable: sanitary products that have been designed to be washed and reused over and over. Some reusable sanitary products can be used for up to 10 years!

A few reminders before you dig deeper into each sanitary option:
- Your body is your private property. No one can touch or photograph you or your sexual organs without your consent. Sexual organs include your breasts, buttocks, and vagina. Tell your parent/guardian or a trusted adult if anyone approaches you or touches you without your consent.
- You should never flush sanitary products!
  - Sanitary products are designed to absorb and some are filled with gels and chemicals that can create blockages in the plumbing if flushed. Always use a sanitary bin to discard used sanitary pads, tampons, and pantyliners!
- *Always* wash your hands before you use the bathroom and touch your vagina.
  - Poor hygiene is the quickest way to getting a pesky and painful infection; see **Her Hygiene** on page 62 on how to care for you and your sanitary products
- Be open minded about reusable products.
  - Our parents didn't have or even know about the plethora of sanitary options available to us today. Although disposable items are convenient, you need to decide for yourself if it's right for you. With the advent of the internet, you can learn more about how to make and use reusable sanitary products.
- Building a Moonbox is fun and easy!
  - Today, sanitary products are easy to buy and customize to suit your mood, clothing, interests! Try mixing and matching different products to find the right protection to suit your flow and style.

External Options

External sanitary products are worn outside the body to **absorb** your menstrual flow. External sanitary products do not go inside the body; instead, they are worn close to the body (inside your underwear). External sanitary options are easy to customize to your favorite fabric, fabric patterns, characters, and size.

External sanitary products are perfect for those who do not wish to use sanitary devices inside the body or may have allergies or sensitivities to materials such as rayon or latex.

Period Panties

Period panties are the best backup protection for sanitary products. Period panties are protective underwear with a waterproof lining to prevent your flow from getting onto your clothes or your bed while you sleep. They are designed to be a comfortable, worry-free garment so you don't need to worry about leaking onto your clothes.

Disposable Period Panties- Always® ZZZ and Kotex U® DreamWear are sold in most stores. Disposable period panties are designed to replace your everyday underwear while you are on your period. Both Always® ZZZ and Kotex U® DreamWear are advertised to keep you leak free while you sleep, whether you are an active or heavy sleeper. Although disposable period underwear is geared to be worn at night, they can be worn at any time during your period. Disposable period underwear is absorbent like a pad, and look kind of like a diaper with stretchy, full coverage material covering your entire bottom from the vagina to your waist. Disposable period underwear come in different sizes to provide you with maximum protection from leaks. Since disposable period underwear gives you complete coverage, you can go about your day and sleep through the night peacefully knowing you're fully protected!

Reusable Period Panties-Reusable period panties continue to grow in popularity due to their unique protection! Period panties come in a variety of colors, styles, and materials to provide you with worry-free protection from leaks. Reusable period panties are worn as your underwear while you are actively flowing on your period. Reusable period panties create a barrier between you and your clothes (or your bed) as the inside layers of material are made with "water-proof" or moisture wicking materials. There are two types of reusable period panties: period panties that are *only* a barrier garment with a PUL (Polyurethane Laminate) or microfiber polyester lining inside the underwear. Barrier period panties are worn with a pad or worn as a backup when using internal sanitary

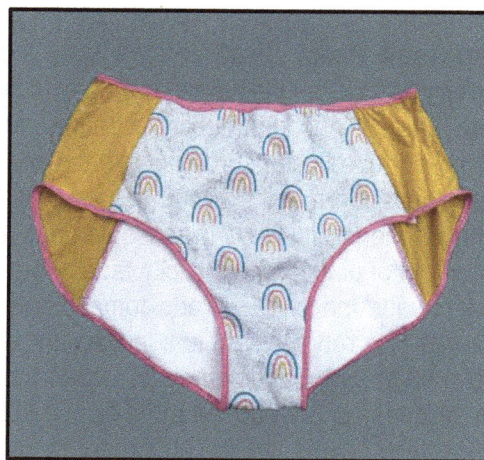

Period Panties made by Liz Carruth
Pattern used with permission from RAD Patterns

options like a tampon or menstrual cup. Specialty period panties, like Unders by Proof®, are period panties with an absorbent core and able to absorb as much fluid as 1-4 tampons. Think of these like a pad sewn into underwear.   Reusable period panties are easy to use as you wear them as a replacement for your daily underwear. To use: slip on over the legs and pull up. If you are wearing period panties with a pad/pantyliner be sure to secure them to the center of the panties before pulling up around the waist. Since period panties are made with various waterproof materials (PUL or microfiber polyester) follow all laundering manufacturer instructions. Although reusable period underwear can be expensive ranging from $10-$30 a pair, reusable period panties are an excellent choice for any menstruating girl's underwear drawer as they are easy to wash, wear, and use again. Reusable period panties will provide many years of quality leak-proof protection. Be sure to wash and care for your investment according to the manufacturer instructions. Reusable period panties can be purchased in some stores but there are a lot of great options online like THINXS®, Cora®, RubyLove®, and Etsy small businesses. For quick shopping, scan the QR code on page 68.

Sanitary Napkins (Pads)

"Sanitary napkins" are the polite name for pads and have a very interesting history! Women have been managing the flow of fluid from their periods since the dawn of time. Sanitary napkins have been made from woven grasses, sheep wool, animal furs, paper, and whatever else women could find that could absorb fluids. Mostly, women have used scraps of fabric or "rags" to absorb their flow which is why some people today still say "I'm on the rag".   It wasn't until 1896 when the first "disposable" pad was designed by French nurses and sold to women. Pads have looked different through the years from rectangular pads of woven fabric to the girdle belt pad women wore in the 1960s. Today, pads are known all around the world by one similar design and are the most common menstrual product for menstruation.

Disposable Pads: Disposable pads are the most common sanitary product available and are easy to find in nearly every store, gas stations, and public restrooms. Pads are elongated tube-like absorbent synthetic and cotton protective liners that adhere to the center of your panties to absorb light to heavy menstrual flow. Disposable pads are wrapped in a thin sheet of plastic with a sticky tape along the back so it can stick to your underwear. Pads come in a variety of absorbances ranging light to super heavy; each absorbance designed to suit your flow needs.   Absorbance will determine the thickness of the pad but most disposable pads are very thin as they have a gel-like absorbent material to absorb your flow. Pads come in a variety of lengths from regular to extra-long. Every girl bleeds differently based on body shape. Some girls find comfort wearing longer pads to make

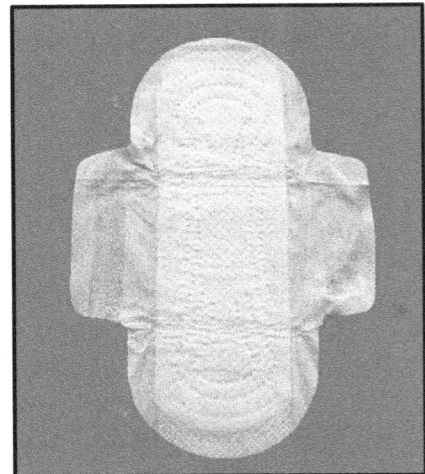

Disposable Sanitary Napkin/Pad
Used with permission from This Is L.

sure they don't leak from the front or back. Some pads have "wings" to fold around the center of the panties to protect from side leakage. To use: remove the outer sheet of plastic and place the pad into the center of the panties ensuring the adhesive has stuck to the panties. It is recommended to change your pads 3-4 hours depending on how fast you are flowing. To remove: simply lift up and pull the pad from the underwear until it is fully removed. Throw the used pad away in the proper sanitary bin next to the toilet. For quick shopping, scan the QR code on page 68.

Reusable Cloth pads: Reusable cloth pads are the original pad and are often referred to in history as "rags". Cloth pads today are much more sophisticated than the long handkerchief-like rags women would wear between their legs to collect their menstrual flow in the *really* old days. Reusable cloth pads look and function just like a store-bought sanitary napkin the only difference is they are reusable and free of chemical absorbent materials. Cloth pads can be as simple or as elaborate as you like! Reusable cloth pads can be made up of your choice of fabric, absorbent material, size, and shape. Since reusable cloth pads are made of natural fibers, cloth pads will decompose faster than store bought pad making them an environmentally friendly choice. Cloth pads can be sewn at home or purchased online from cloth pad retailers such as Glad Rags® or cloth pad makers on Etsy®, Amazon®, or local sewers. Cloth pads tend to be thicker than store bought pads but the design is similar. Reusable cloth pads are elongated tube-like fabric liners made of sewn layers of absorbent

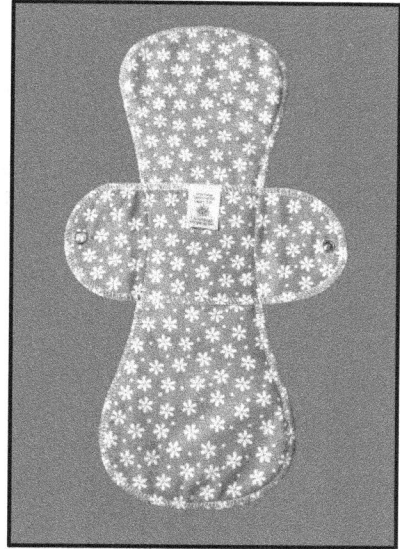

Reusable Sanitary Napkin/Pad
Used with permission from Gland Rags

materials and sewn together into the shape of a pad. Reusable cloth pads can also come with or without wings. There are a large variety of shapes and lengths to accommodate different body types, style, and flow. Examples of some fun shapes are cats, teddy bears, vampires, and crowns. To use: simply place the cloth pad into the center of the panties and pull your underwear up. If your cloth pad has wings, be sure to secure it around the center of your panties. It is recommended to change your pad every 3-4 hours depending on how fast you are flowing. To change your pad: simply lift up and remove the used pad and place in a "wet bag*" or another storage bag of your choice to bring home to wash. After your period has stopped flowing, wash ALL of the soiled pads according to the manufacturer's instructions. Once they are washed and dry, put away until you need them next month. For further details regarding washing and storing of reusable cloth pads see **Her Hygiene** page 62.

Pantyliners

Pantyliners are the little sister to the pad. Typically, pantyliners are much thinner and shorter because they are used for light to extremely light flow, like when you are **spotting** (a very light bleeding) or ending your period, or as backup protection to an internal sanitary device like a tampon or menstrual cup. Pantyliners are worn when menstrual fluid is not flowing enough to wear a pad but there is enough of it to need protection from wetness and staining of your underwear.

Disposable Pantyliners: Disposable pantyliners are extremely thin oblong absorbent synthetic and cotton protective liners that you adhere to the center of your panties to absorb menstrual fluid. Disposable pantyliners also come in a variety of absorbances and lengths to suit your body shape and flow. Some pantyliners come scented, use cautiously as scents are made with synthetic chemicals that can irritate the delicate skin of the vagina causing itching and rashes. To use: remove the outer sheet of plastic and place it into the center of the panties. To change your pantyliner: lift the liner from the panties and throw it away in the proper sanitary bin next to the toilet. It is recommended to change your pad every 3-4 hours but typically with a liner you should only need to change it once or twice a day.

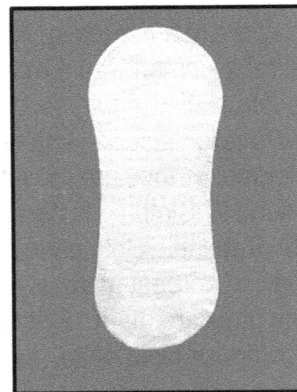

Disposable Pantyliner
Used with permission from This Is L.

Reusable Cotton Pantyliners: Reusable cloth pantyliners look and function just like a store-bought pantyliner only they are reusable and free of chemical absorbent materials. Reusable cloth pantyliners are light layers of fabric cut into an oblong shape and sewn in the shape of a pantyliner. Just like cloth pads, reusable cloth pantyliners can be made from your choice of fabric, absorbent material, size, and shape. To use: simply place it into the center of the panties and pull up your underwear. If your cloth pad has wings, be sure to secure around the center of your panties to keep it from moving around. When your pantyliner has become soiled and needs to be changed: simply lift up, remove the used pantyliner, and place into a "wet bag*" or another storage bag of your choice to bring home to wash. It is recommended to change your pad every 3-4 hours but typically with a pantyliner you should only need to change it once or twice a day. Always wash your stash of cloth pantyliners after each use and store in a clean bag or bin until you are ready to use them again. For quick shopping, scan the QR code on page 68.

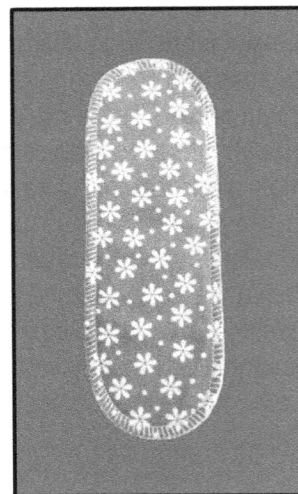

Reusable Pantyliner
Used with permission from Glad Rags

Interlabia Pads

Interlabia pads: Interlabia pads are unique, and not well known, but they serve your menstrual flow similar to a pantyliner. Instead of wearing the liner inside the underwear, you place the interlabia pad between the lips of the vagina (also known as the **labia**). The folds of the labia hold the pad against the vagina. Interlabia pads are like a miniature cloth pantyliner, typically "leaf" shaped, that can be used on its own for very light flow or as an additional layer to absorb heavy flow. Interlabia pads fold down along its center as a leaf would along its stem and remain in place when the lips of the vagina close around the fabric. To use: place the leaf shaped pad against the vaginal opening, allowing the labia to fold the interlabia pad in half. The pad should lie against the walls of the labia and cover the vaginal opening to absorb fluid. When the interlabia pad is wet or soiled with menstrual fluid it will need to be changed. To change: simply remove the interlabia pad from between the labia and place it into a wet bag or another storage bag of your

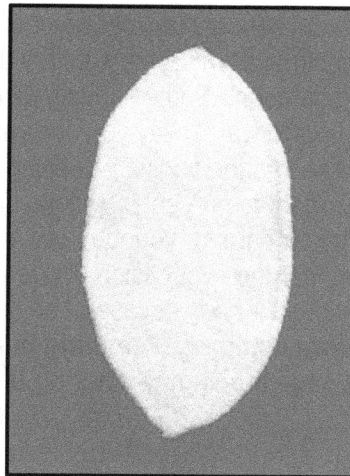

Reusable Interlabia Pad
Used with permission from EcoAdorable

choice to bring home to wash. It is recommended to change your pad every 3-4 hours depending on how fast you are flowing, especially if you are using the interlabia pad to collect heavy flow. If you are using the interlabia pad on light days, you should replace the used interlabia pad with a clean interlaiba pad often since it sits at the vagina opening and will be moist. Always wash your stash of interlabia pads after use and store in a clean bag or bin until you are ready to use them again. Interlabia pads are not found in stores but are sold through cloth pad businesses such as EcoAdorble® or Etsy shops. For quick shopping, scan the QR code on page 68.

Internal Options

Internal sanitary devices are worn *inside* your body (inside the vagina) to collect or absorb your menstrual flow. Some sanitary devices come with applicators to insert devices into your vagina, such as a tampon. Some sanitary devices are inserted with your hand (digital insertion). **Digital insertion** is a polite way to say you use your hands and your "digits" (fingers) to insert and remove a sanitary device into the vagina. Keeping your internal sanitary devices clean and sanitized is extremely important to prevent infections in and around your vagina. Please refer to **Her Hygiene** on page 62 to better care for your devices and body. Always use internal sanitary devices with the permission of, or under the supervision of a responsible adult so they are aware that you have a medical device inside your body in case of an emergency. **Speak to your parents/guardian or trusted adult before using or attempting to use an internal sanitary device. Using the wrong size can damage the vagina causing tears and pain.**

Tampons

Tampons are "tubes" of tightly woven or wound material that are inserted into the vagina to collect menstrual fluid. Tampon-like solutions for managing menstrual flow have been used around the world for a very long time and made from a variety of materials such as rolled rice paper, papyrus, and even wooden tampons. It wasn't until the 1960's that the more recognizable tampon we use today was invented. Like menstrual pads, tampons have taken different shapes over the years but they still function by absorbing menstrual fluid from inside the vagina.

Disposable Tampons: Disposable tampons are a woven cotton tube (sometimes synthetic materials like rayon) that is inserted into your vagina to absorb menstrual fluid. Tampons come in absorbances (sizes): light, medium, super, and extra super. Choosing an absorbance depends on where you are at in your period. Generally, your period will start with a heavy flow until it slows down to light discharge. Tampons swell as they absorb so be sure to pick the correct size. Tampons are pre-packaged with a one-time use applicator made of plastic or cardboard to aid in the insertion of the tampon. Only **one** tampon is worn at a time. Always **remove** the used tampon before inserting a new one. To use: open the packaging and extend the applicator. Insert gently into your vagina and press the plunger to release the tampon. Remove the applicator from your vagina and throw it away in the sanitary bin next to the toilet. The string of the tampon should be felt outside of the vagina. Tampons should be changed every 3-4 hours or until full. To remove, gently pull

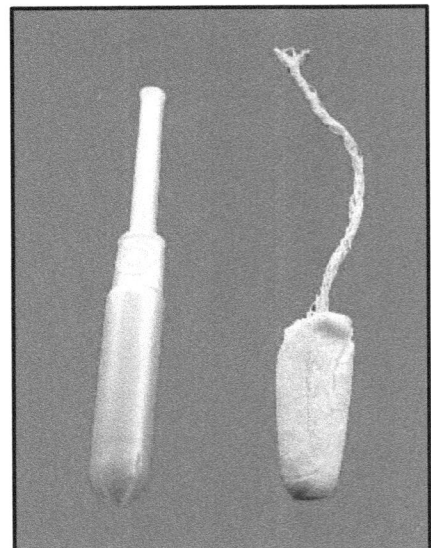

Disposable Tampon
Used with permission from This is L.

the string until the tampon falls away from your vagina and throw it away in a sanitary bin. It is a good idea to wear a pantyliner or pad as a backup in case your tampon leaks from being too full or inserted incorrectly. Period panties also make an excellent back up to a tampon. Tampons are a great tool for sports and swimming as it allows you to absorb your flow and continue doing the things you love. For quick shopping, scan the QR code on page 68.

Reusable Tampons: Reusable tampons come in a lot of different styles from crochet to fabric. Reusable tampons are usually made from a very thin material and rolled tightly into a 1-inch tube to insert into the vagina to absorb your menstrual fluid. Reusable tampon absorbances are determined by how long the tampon roll is. The longer the fabric of the tampon, the thicker (more absorbent) the tampon will be. Always make sure the string end of the tampon is on the outside of the rolled tube. If you choose to use reusable tampons, you can find reusable tampon applicators online through vendors such as eBay® or Amazon® to make the insertion to the vagina much easier or you can **reuse** a disposable plastic applicator to insert your reusable tampon. To use: roll the tampon very tightly into a 1-inch tube, ensuring the string is facing the bottom of the tampon. Place the rolled tampon into the applicator and insert into your vagina. The string of the tampon should be felt outside of your vagina. Tug gently to make sure the reusable tampon is secured in place. When the string is tugged the tampon should not fall out or move around. Tampons should be changed every 3-4 hours or when full. To remove: gently pull on the string until the tampon comes out of your vagina and place it into a wet bag or another bag of your choice to bring home to wash. It is always a good idea to wear a pad or pantyliner as a backup in case your tampon leaks from being too full or inserted incorrectly. Always wash your reusable tampons when your period is finished and store clean tampons in a bag or bin until your next period. Reusable tampon applicators can be washed in a bowl of warm water and gentle soap inside and out or according to the manufacturer's instructions.

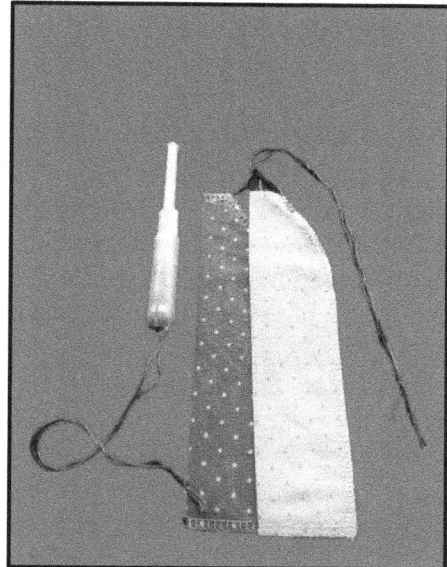

Reusable Fabric Tampon with Applicator
Used with permission from Liz Carruth

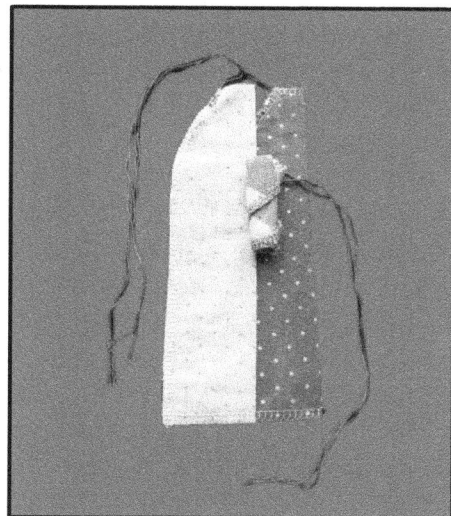

Reusable Fabric Rolled to Insert
Used with permission from Liz Carruth

Menstrual Discs

Menstrual discs are round ring-like collection bags for menstrual fluid that is worn inside the vagina. Menstrual discs are definitely worth a try as they can be worn for up to 12 hours! That's a half a day, mostly, period-free! Menstrual discs are held in place behind the pubic bone so learning to insert and remove properly takes some *practice* so don't be discouraged when you don't get it right the first time. For quick shopping, scan the QR code on page 68.

Disposable Menstrual Discs: Flex® and Softdisc® disposables are round plastic rings with a very thin plastic collection bag that you fold and insert into your vagina to collect menstrual fluids. Only one menstrual disc is used at a time and thrown away after it is used. Disposable menstrual discs are like a cross between a disposable tampon and a menstrual cup; discs *collect* rather than absorb so removal can be messy. Disposable menstrual discs are designed to be worn longer than a tampon (up to 12 hours) and collect more fluid than your traditional tampon. However, there is one drawback for newer menstruating girls: they do not come in small sizes, only "one size fits all." Disposable menstrual discs take some practice to get the hang of using, as the folding and inserting take some practice to get into place behind the public bone just right. You should check with an adult before trying disposable menstrual discs as they are designed for older women who have larger vaginas and have more experience inserting and removing sanitary devices from their vaginas. Always read manufacturing instructions. To insert: fold sides in half and gently push inside until you feel it expand. The disc will sit right behind the pubic bone and hold it in place. Disposable menstrual discs are designed to be worn for up to 12 hours so you will have to learn when it feels "full" or you begin to leak. To remove: while sitting on the toilet, insert a clean finger into your vagina and loop your finger around the rim and gently pull the disc out until it is removed. You will need to pour out the fluid into the toilet and discard into the proper sanitary bin next to the toilet. It is a good idea to wear a pantyliner or pad as a backup in case your menstrual disc leaks from being too full or inserted incorrectly. Removing a disposable menstrual disc can be messy but worth it if you want hours of period protection.

Reusable Menstrual Discs: Like disposable menstrual discs but built to last! Reusable menstrual discs are round silicone rings with a thin silicon collection bag that you fold and insert into the vagina to collect menstrual fluids. Unlike disposable menstrual discs, a well-cared for reusable menstrual disc can be used for many years providing you with many years of earth-friendly menstrual care. Menstrual discs take some practice to get the hang of using, as the folding and inserting take some practice to get into place behind the public bone just right. Reusable menstrual discs are designed to be worn longer than a tampon (up to 12 hours) as they have the ability to collect more fluid than your traditional tampon. Some reusable discs have a grabbing "notch" or tether to aid in the easy insertion and removal of menstrual discs.

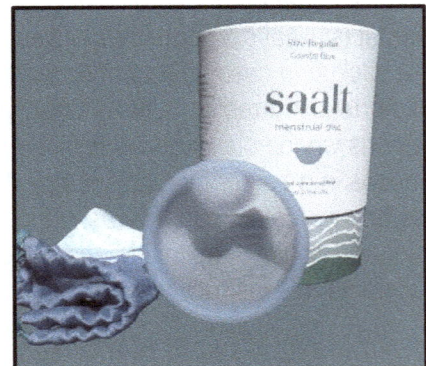

Reusable Menstrual Disc
Used with permission from Saalt

Like menstrual cups, reusable menstrual discs come in sizes: small and large. "Large" reusable menstrual discs have been designed for older women who have larger vaginas and/or have had a baby so a "large" disc won't fit young girls comfortably. Even "small" menstrual discs may be too large for a new menstruating girl so you should check with an adult before trying a reusable menstrual disc. To insert: fold sides in half and gently push inside until you feel it expand. The disc will sit right behind the public bone and hold it in place. Reusable menstrual discs are designed to be worn for up to 12 hours so you will have to learn when it feels "full" or you begin to leak. It is always a good idea to wear a pantyliner or pad as a backup in case your menstrual disc leaks from being too full or inserted incorrectly. To remove: while sitting on the toilet, insert a clean finger into the vagina and loop your finger around the rim or gasp the notch and gently pull out the disc until it is removed from your vagina. Pour out the fluid into the toilet and wash the reusable menstrual disc with warm water to reinsert. You should sanitize your menstrual disc daily to disinfect. Your reusable menstrual disc will need to be sterilized before storing. For detailed information on sanitizing your menstrual disc, see "**Her Hygiene**" page 62.

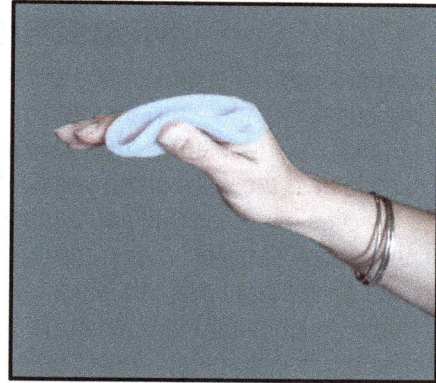

Folded Saalt Disc for Insertion
Used with permission from Saalt
Modeled by: Rebecca Clawson

Menstrual Cups

Menstrual Cups: Menstrual cups are a little bell-shaped silicone cup with a stem and inserted into the vagina to collect menstrual fluids. Menstrual cups have little holes around the rim to suction to the walls of the vagina. Menstrual cups take some practice to get the hang of but they are an earth-friendly, reusable option to collect menstrual fluid. If used and stored property, a menstrual cup can last a few years making it an affordable option at $10-$20 a cup. To insert: fold according to manufacturer's instructions, insert, wait for it to unfold and suction against the vaginal walls. "Tug Test " to ensure it has suctioned against the vagina walls by gently tugging the stem to make sure it is secured in place. If inserted properly, when the stem is tugged on you should feel it pull, not move or slip. Menstrual cups come in 2 sizes: small and large (large are for women over 30 or who have had a child). Size matters so double check that you are using the correct size to collect your flow. Menstrual cups are designed to be worn for up to 12 hours but depending on your flow it may need to be emptied sooner. It is always a good idea to wear a pantyliner or pad as a backup in case your menstrual cup leaks from being too full or inserted incorrectly. Before you insert the cup for the first time, practice the manufacturer's folding technique. Notice how the cup opens when released and note how it feels when it opens. The most common folding technique is the "C" fold, but if you have trouble with one technique don't be afraid to try another. YouTube has demonstration videos on the various techniques to fold and insert menstrual cups. To remove: with a clean hand reach into the vagina and with the index finger and thumb pull on the stem until the cup is removed.

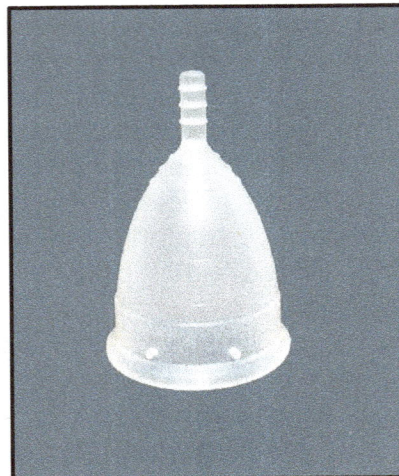

Lunette Menstrual Cup
Used with permission from Lunette

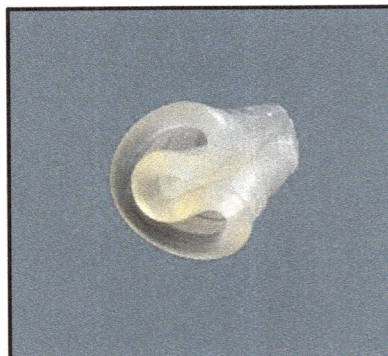

"C" fold of Lunette Cup
Used with permission from Lunette

Wash well with warm water and reinsert. You should aim to sanitize once a day with boiling water to keep your vagina clean of bacteria. Your cup should be deep cleaned and sanitized before storing until your next period. To sanitize: using a pot/bowl place the menstrual cup into boiling water for 3-5 minutes. Dry and place into the storage bag to use for your next period. Menstrual cups are a great tool for sports and swimming as it allows you to collect your fluids and continue doing the things you love. For quick shopping, scan the QR code on page 68.

Sea Sponges

Sea Sponges: Sea Sponges are the *only* 100% natural way to absorb your flow. Sea Sponges have been used as far back as ancient times for menstrual care. Rumor has it that Egyptian Queen Cleopatra used sea sponges for her menstrual flow! Natural sea sponges are harvested from the sea and are washed, inspected, and sold to small market vendors who trim and package the sea sponges to sell as for feminine care. Since sea sponges are inherently absorbent, they are the safest choice for menstrual care as they are not manufactured or processed by any other means than the sea. Sea Sponges are like a tampon, only 100% natural. Sea Sponges are inserted into the vagina (one or two at a time) to absorb menstrual fluid. Sea Sponges, like the ones sold by Jade and Pearls® come in a 2 pack and variety of sizes (absorbency): teeny, small, medium, large, and multipack (one of each). Sea Sponges provide you the flexibility to absorb your flow according to your body's needs. Jade and Pearl made a teen size one for smaller vaginas. You can wear both sponges at once or as your flow lightens up, one at a time. Sea Sponges are able to be worn and reused after rinsing every 3-4 hours and are safe to use overnight up to 8 hours. Sea Sponges are also completely customizable to your body's shape as you can trim the sponge to fit your needs. Sea Sponges are delicate but a well-cared for sponge can last up to a year or more and is a renewable source! Sea Sponges need to be cleaned before using them for the first time; be sure to follow all manufacturer's instructions of how to properly clean your sea sponges to get the best and longest use possible. To use: wet the sponge until it is saturated, squeeze out excess water, and gently push one sponge into the vagina at a time.

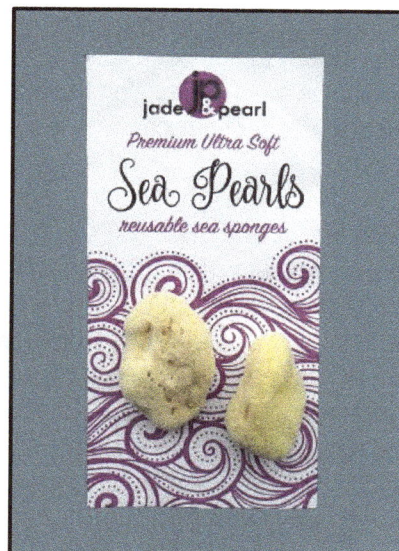

Reusable Sea Pearl "Tampon"
Used with permission from Jade & Pearls

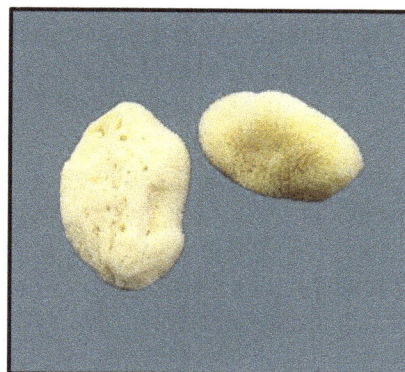

Reusable Sea Pearl
Used with permission from Jade & Pearls

The sponge should feel secure and comfortable. To remove, feel for the edge of the sponge and grasp it gently. Pull the sea sponge until it comes out of your vagina (repeat if you are using two at a time). Sea Sponges do not need to be sanitized between uses so rinse with water and reinsert. It is always a good idea to wear a pantyliner or pad as a backup in case your sea sponge leaks from being too full. Sanitize your sea sponges according to the manufacturer instructions, allow them to fully dry, and store them until your next period. Jade and Pearl provide 4 safe sanitizing options to use with their all-natural Sea Sponges. For quick shopping, scan the QR code on page 68.

Just for Tweens & Teens

Tweens and Teens have smaller bodies than adults making some really affordable and reusable items harder to use because they have been designed for grown women to use. Luckily, some companies have recognized the gap between adult and teen needs and have produced some reusable sanitary devices with tween and teen girls in mind! For quick shopping, scan the QR code on page 68.

TEEN Menstrual disc: Currently, there is only *one* menstrual disc designed for teen girls ages 11 and older. The "PrettiPersonal" Menstrual Disc is *perfectly* sized for tweens and teenage girls who are comfortable with inserting and removing sanitary devices from the vagina (digital insertion). The PrettiPersonal® disc is a hybrid of disposable and reusable menstrual discs. PrettiPersonal® disc is made from 100% medical grade silicone and is reusable up to three menstrual cycles!

For more information on menstrual discs and how to use them see page 56.

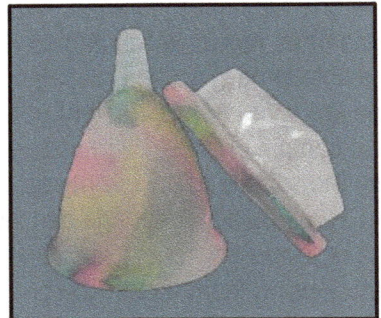

"PrettiPersonal" Teen Menstrual Disc
Used with permission from PrettiPersonal

TEEN Menstrual cups: GladRags® XO Flo Mini®, June Cup Mini®, Lunette® model 1, Pixie Cup Teen®, PrettiPersonal® Teen menstrual cup, and Saalt® Teen Cup are just a few trusted brands that sell cups designed for young tween/ teenage girls. Each company has thorough details regarding their cup, how its designed for teenagers, cup folding guides, videos of how to use and care for your menstrual cup. Do some research and find the right cup for you!

For a detailed explanation of menstrual cups see page 58.

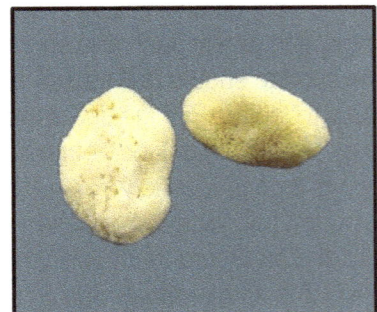

"PrettiPersonal Teen Menstrual cup
Used with permission from PrettiPersonal

TEEN Sea Sponge: Jade and Pearls® "Teeny" size Sea Sponges and Glad Rags®.
For full details on sea sponges see page 59.

TEEN Period Panties: Thinx® BTWEEN, "KT" by Knixteen®, RubyLove® Teen underwear (and swimwear bottoms), Etsy® period panty shops.
For full details on period panties on page 49.

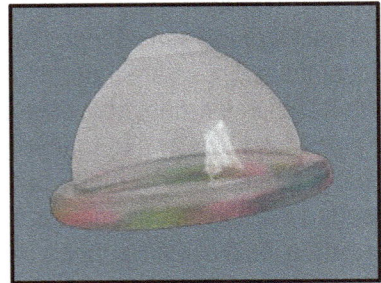

Reusable Sea Pearls
Used with permission from Jade & Pearl

Her Hygiene

Hygiene is the number one priority when it comes to your body, especially when you're on your period! **Hygiene** is the daily practice of keeping the body clean through bathing, hand washing, frequently changing sanitary products, and daily changing of clothes. The products on this list are not essential to maintaining your menstrual flow. They are "feel-good" products to help manage your period and keep you feeling fresh!

Do become familiar with reading product packaging and become familiar with the ingredients to know what is or isn't safe for the vagina. The vagina has a very delicate ecosystem (a biological community of microbes and organisms that connect together to maintain a balanced environment).   Special soaps, lotions, creams have been created with the vaginal ecosystem in mind. These products are perfectly balanced to maintain your vaginas natural balance. If you choose to use anything other than soap and water, be sure to read the label or try to choose dye and perfume free products.

Disposable Feminine wipes- Disposable feminine wipes are like a baby wipe but made with a vaginal pH balancing solution. Disposable feminine wipes are convenient to carry in your purse, backpack, or wet bag so you can freshen up after you use the bathroom. To use: remove the wipe from its pouch and wipe from front to back, across your vagina, inside and outside of the labia, and folds of the groin. Place the used disposable feminine wipe into the sanitary bin next to the toilet. Disposable feminine wipes can be found in individually wrapped packages to carry discreetly in your pocket or purse.

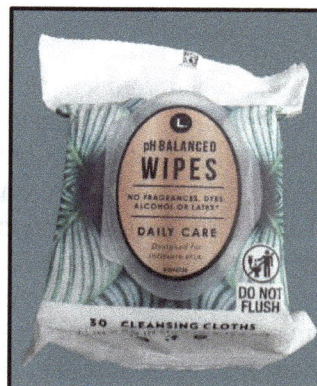

Disposable Feminine Wipe
Used with permission from This Is L.

Reusable Feminine wipes- Reusable feminine wipes are typically made from flannel cotton fabric and cut into palm size squares to be used in a solution of water, witch hazel, and castile soap to wash up between bathing. Reusable feminine wipes can be used even when you're not on your period, you can use the reusable feminine wipes to freshen up after sports or on hot days, really anytime you feel the need to freshen up. Since reusable feminine wipes are made with gentle ingredients, you can use them all over the body! Just be sure to use a trusted solution recipe with ingredients that are vagina safe and with adult supervision. To use: remove the wipe from its container and wipe from front to back, across your vagina, inside and outside of the labia, and folds of the groin. Place the used cotton wipe into a wet bag along with any soiled pad/pantyliners

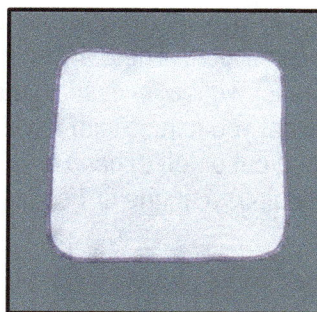

Reusable Feminine Wipe
Used with permission from Liz Carruth

and wash with your period sanitary items. Reusable feminine wipes can be stored in a zipper baggie, reusable baby wipe box, travel baby wipe container/bag/pouch. Reusable cotton wipes and containers can be purchased fairly cheaply and easily through retailers such as Amazon®, Etsy, and some baby diapering companies. For quick shopping, scan the QR code on page 68!

Feminine Wash-Perfectly formulated soap to be used specifically on the female body, the vagina. Feminine wash has been tested for the vaginal area so it does not create any dryness, irritation, or rashes. Feminine wash comes ready to use in a foam or liquid bottle that you simply apply to a washcloth or loofah and wash your groin area (this includes your vagina and buttocks). While there are feminine washes designed to be specifically used during your period, most feminine washes are safe for daily use. Be sure to read the label and follow all manufacturer instructions.

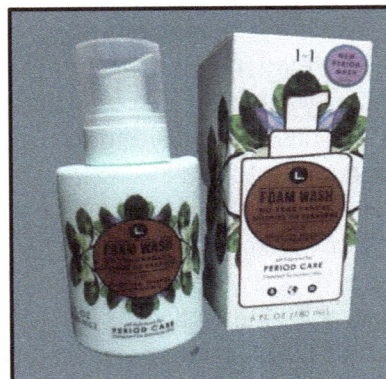

Feminine Wash
Used with permission from This Is L.

Wet Bag-A waterproof, leak resistant bag or pouch to store your used pads/pantyliners in so it doesn't get menstrual fluid in your pocket, purse, or backpack. Wet bags can be made from PUL, Oil Cloth, vinyl, laminated cotton/canvas, or fleece. We bags are very customizable with fabric of your choice or though small businesses such as Hem and Haw on Etsy. Wet bags come in a variety of closures from zippers, snaps, and drawstrings. Wet bags come in a variety of sizes from pocket zipper bags to large bags you can clip onto your toilet paper holder to hold all your pads until you are ready to wash them. You can find some wet bags in local stores and online, near baby items or in the travel section. There are so many types of styles and

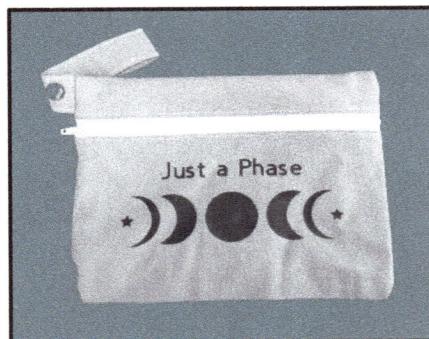

"Zipper" Wet Bag with Purse Snap
Used with permission from HemandHaw

uses for wet bags, even if you're not using reusable menstrual products, your imagination is the limit to what you can do with a wet bag. NOTE: Wet bags are usually not washed aggressively, just wiped out or left to hang dry. Be sure to follow all manufacturing laundering instructions. For quick shopping, scan the QR code on page 68!

Storing and Cleaning Reusable Sanitary Products

There are two ways to store your soiled (used/dirty) pads as you go through your period: "dry" storage and "wet" storage. Both are temporary ways to contain your used sanitary items until you wash *all* of your sanitary items at the end of your period.

During your Period Storage

Dry storage- Placing all your soiled pads in a bag or bucket until you are ready to wash them all together. Dry storage means you do not wash or rinse the menstrual fluid off of the pad/pantyliners after you soil them. The pads/pantyliners go into the storage container in the condition you remove them from your underwear. The pads/pantyliners dry out until you're ready to wash all of your menstrual items at one time. One problem with dry storage is staining. Staining won't affect the usefulness of the pads/pantyliners but can make them less attractive. Stains are usually preventable with immediate gentle care such as rinsing and wringing the pads out. If you choose to dry store your pads through your period, you may need to soak your pads/pantyliners before washing in a washing machine to get the majority of the dried fluid soft enough to wash away. * There are a couple of specialty items you can purchase to make dry storage a breeze. There are wet bags that come in a variety of shapes and sizes: toilet roll clip on bags, trash bag liners that turn into a wet bag, a simple bucket or tote, laundry bag, or mesh zipper bags are just a few ways you can store your soiled sanitary pads/pantyliners until you are ready to wash them. Your storage container doesn't have to be elaborate or expensive, just functional.

*Never rinse and dry store your pads. Rinsed pads need to be washed immediately or use the wet storage technique.

Wet storage-Placing all of your soiled pads in a bucket of water until your period is over to wash all your menstrual items together. The water will turn bright red as the menstrual fluid seeps from the soiled pads and into the water. It is best to have a dedicated plastic trash can, bucket, or tote devoted to the wet storage of your pads/pantyliners so no one uses it for any other purpose. When you are ready to wash all of your menstrual items you will need to dump the wet pads out in the tub or fish them out to place into the washing machine. The "wet" storage method is used to prevent staining your pads and pantyliners. Adding hydrogen peroxide to your bucket of water will help keep the light colors vibrant and prevent the iron in the blood from sticking to the fabric causing stains.

Cleaning

Some choose to clean their pads right away by washing off the pads/pantyliner with a shower head or in the sink until the water from the pad runs clear. Some choose to throw their pads from the day in with a load of laundry and wash their sanitary items as they use them (this method does not require wet or dry storage). Another cleaning option would be to wash them by hand with soap and water or you can wash them with a washboard. The easiest method to pre-clean your solid pads (from wet or dry storage) is to "stomp" them clean while taking a shower. The **stomp** method is a brilliant way to reuse water and "kill two birds with one stone" by taking a shower and cleaning your pads at the same time. To "stomp" your pads: take all of your soiled pads and place them into the bottom of the tub or shower and let the water run over them. As you climb in the shower to bathe, walk back and forth, march, and mash the pads with your feet (your feet will become the power source to remove embedded fluid from the pad similar to the tumbling and agitation from a washing machine). As you wash up, let the soap fall freely onto the pads below and continue to "stomp" the pads. By the time you are finished showering, your pads should have most of the fluid washed away and clear water flowing through the pads. Wring out excess water and place all the pads/pantyliners into the washing machine to wash. You can incorporate the "stomp" method into your daily bathing routine while you're on your period or you can choose to "stomp" all of your soiled sanitary items at one time before you put them into the washing machine. If you choose to use dry storage, only "stomp" the pads clean when you are ready to wash all of your pads at the end of your period. Do not rinse or stomp your pad/pantyliners and then place wet pads in dry storage. You will cause the pad to become unusable due to mold and bacteria will settle into your pads while you wait to wash them all. In conclusion, it does not matter which way you choose to clean your pads, just be sure to wash them by the manufacturer's instructions so you can enjoy your reusable pads for many periods to come!

In Between Storage

Storage can be tricky if you build too large of a reusable menstrual product stash. Luckily, there are a lot of creative ways to put your sanitary products away until your next period. Some choose to store pads in their dresser draw along with their underwear. Some choose to store their sanitary products in a bin or tote or bag under the bathroom sink or in the linen closet. Some choose to keep it simple and have only as many sanitary products as necessary. Your favorite retail stores and websites are sure to have a containment solution for all of your products, it's totally up to you what kind of method you choose to store your sanitary products. The bottom line of sanitary product storage: make sure your sanitary products are *clean* and *dry before* storing them away. Each product will have its own cleaning and storage instructions. Menstrual cups and discs recommend boiling the cup/disc prior to storing it away until your next period. Sea Sponges require sanitizing and drying before storing them until your next period. Cloth pads and pantyliners require a thorough wash with a washing machine. Become familiar with your sanitary products and how they are to be cleaned, also which cleaning products are safe for the materials in your sanitary products.

Cleaning and Sanitizing Menstrual Cups and Discs

Internal sanitary devices, such as menstrual cups and discs, need to be washed each day while you are on your period. Daily washing can be accomplished while in the shower, at your bathroom sink, or performed between changing your pad. It is recommended to wash your internal sanitary device with a gentle soap and warm water. Some internal sanitary device companies offer cup/disc wash approved to be used with their product but regular soap and water will also do the job just fine.

At the end of your period when you no longer require an internal sanitary device, you must sanitize your internal sanitary device. Sanitizing can be accomplished a few different ways by boiling your menstrual cup or disc in a pot of boiling water or placing the cup/disc into a bowl of boiling water. It is not recommended to microwave your cup/disc inside the microwave. It is safe to water that has been heated from a microwave but do not place your cup or disc into the microwave and turn it on to boil inside the microwave. You will ruin your menstrual cup/disc.

Sanitizing luxuries

Luxuries do not mean unaffordable! The listed sanitizing luxuries below are not necessities for menstruating. The items listed below are for your awareness and consideration as an investment to making your menstrual cycle each month even easier. There are many sanitizing options available to deep clean (sanitize) your internal sanitary devices.

Sanitizing Cup Wash- Most menstrual cup/disc companies have their own "cup/disc" wash (soap solution) to sanitize your cup after your period. Sanitizing solutions are meant to remove any residue, staining and buildup on your menstrual cup. Menstrual cup/disc sanitizing washes are specifically designed not to erode or deteriorate the materials of your sanitary devices as well as being perfectly balanced to use inside the vagina. A few notable companies have their own cup wash: Saalt® Cup Wash, Pixie Cup® Menstrual Cup Wash, Cora®, Honeypot®, Lunette® "Feel better" Cup cleanser. Use according to the instructions on the label.

Collapsible Sterilizing Cup- The collapsible sterilizing cup has been designed to be taken with you to sterilize or wash your menstrual cup/disc while in public restrooms. The sterilizing cup folds down around itself making it small enough to fit in your purse or backpack. To use: open the sterilizing cup and fill with hot water. After removing the cup/disc from the vagina and emptying into the toilet, drop the cup/disc into the hot water and let it sit in the hot water before reinserting into the vagina. You can also utilize the sterilizing cup to sterilize your cup/disc for end of period storage by filling the cup with boiling water and letting it sit for 3 minutes in the boiling water. Most collapsible sterilizing cups are under $10 and can be found on some

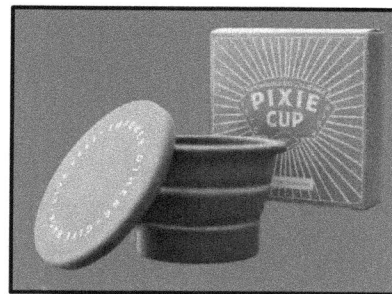

Collapsible Sterilizing Cup
Used with permission from Pixie Cup

menstrual cup/disc webpages with their products such as Pixie Cup®, Amazon®, Wish®, and other retailers.

Menstrual cup/disc steamer or UV light sanitizer-
An electric device that has a chamber to place your
menstrual cup/disc into it and where it will use steam to
sterilize the cup/disc. There are also electric devices just like
the menstrual cup/disc steamer that use UV light to sanitize
your menstrual products. Both of these sterilizing devices are
pretty neat and cost just under $30 on Amazon®. To use:
place a capful of bottled water into the sterilizing chamber
and place your cup/disc over the steaming vent. Secure the
steaming chamber and press the ON button. Most steamers
come with an automatic timer but if it does not have a timer
be sure to watch the clock so you know when your cup/disc
is finished sterilizing. Let the cup/disc cool before
reinserting. The benefit of having a dedicated device is that
you can use it discreetly so you don't need to use the family

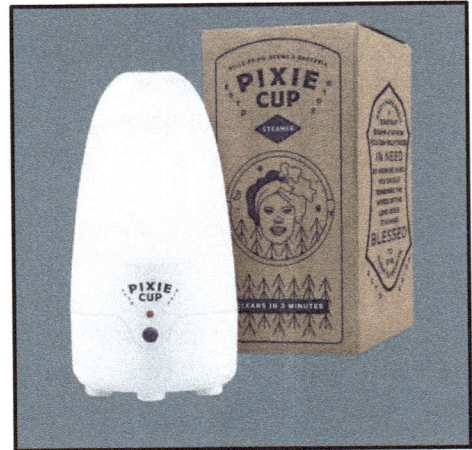

Menstrual Cup/Disc Steamer
Used with permission from Pixie Cup

kitchen space and cookware to sterilize your menstrual cup/disc you can use it in the privacy of your
own bathroom. Menstrual cup/disc sanitizers can be found at Pixie Cup®, Amazon®, and Walmart®
online. For quick shopping, scan the QR code on page 68!

Index

Anemia-An iron deficiency caused by lack of red blood cells

Anatomy-The study of the inner workings of something (i.e. human body)

External-Outside your body

Fallopian Tube-Both pair of tubes along which an egg travels from the ovaries to the uterus

Genitalia–The word that describes the external parts of the female reproductive system.

Groin-The area between the abdomen and the thigh; (the crease where your leg and vulva meet)

Hormones-The invisible chemicals inside our body that tell parts of our body how to work.

Hygiene-Practice of maintaining health and preventing disease through cleanliness

Internal-Inside your body

Labia-Outer folds of the female genitalia

Menses-Blood and lining discharged from the uterus at menstruation

Menstruation-Process by which women discharge blood and lining from the uterus each month

Ovary-Female reproductive organ in which eggs are produced

Ovulation-Releasing of an egg from the ovary

Period-Anther word to say "menstruation"

PMS-**PreMenstrual Syndrome** refers to the complex symptoms experienced before menstruation

Private-A polite way to refer to your sex organs, also known as your vagina or genitalia

Puberty- The process by which your body makes *physical* changes to become an adult

Sanitary-The conditions that affect hygiene and health

Sanitize-To make something clean and hygienic; disinfected

Soiled-Dirty or used

Uterus-Female reproductive organ of where a child is conceived and grown until it is born

Vagina-Muscular tube leading from the external genitals to the cervix of the uterus

Vulva-The female external genitals

Sources

Background Remover
https://www.remove.bg

CDC
https://www.cdc.gov/ncbddd/blooddisorders/women/menorrhagia.html

Femme International "History of Sanitary Pad"
https://femmeinternational.org/the-history-of-the-sanitary-pad/

Fibroid Specialists
https://www.fibroidspecialists.org/post/fibroid-cyst-polyp

John Hopkins Medicine
https://hopkinsmedicine.org/health/wellness-and-prevention/menstrual-cycle-an-overview

Kids Health
https://kidshealth.org/en/teens/menstrual-problems.html

Mayo Clinic
https://www.mayoclinic.org/healthy-lifestyle/womens-health/in-depth/menstrual-cycle/art-20047186

Nationwide Childrens
https://www.nationwidechildrens.org/family-resources-education/health-wellness-and-safety-resources/helping-hands/body-system-reproductive-female

Nutritionist Resource
https://www.nutritionist-resource.org.uk/memberarticles/what-foods-give-a-menstruating-woman-energy

OB/GYN Specialists
https://www.pro-lifeobgyn.com/blog/can-heavy-periods-cause-anemia

Oxford Languages
https://languages.oup.com/dictionaries/

Pratisandhi
https://www.pratisandhi.com/menstruation-euphemisms/

Rael "When were Tampons Invented? A Brief History of Tampons"
https://www.getrael.com/blogs/r-blog/when-were-tampons-invented
Stanford Children's Health
https://www.stanfordchildrens.org/en/topic/default?id=menstrual-cycle-an-overview-85-P00553

Tampax*   *Direct quotes were used with permission from Proctor and Gamble and Tampax
https://tampax.com/en-us/tampon-truths/do-tampons-take-your-virginity/
https://tampax.com/en-us/period-health/toxic-shock-syndrome-causes-treatment/

www.ingramcontent.com/pod-product-compliance
Lightning Source LLC
Chambersburg PA
CBHW081721270326
41933CB00017B/3254